# Recent Results in Cancer Research 58

Fortschritte der Krebsforschung
Progrès dans les recherches sur le cancer

Bruce S. Schoenberg

# Multiple Primary Malignant Neoplasms

## The Connecticut Experience, 1935-1964

In collaboration with
B. W. Christine J. F. Fraumeni, Jr.
R. A. Greenberg D. G. Schoenberg

With 139 Tables

Springer-Verlag
Berlin Heidelberg New York 1977

Bruce S. Schoenberg, M.D., M.P.H. in Epidemiology, M.S. in Neurology, Visiting Scientist, Department of Medical Statistics and Epidemiology and Department of Neurology, Mayo Clinic, Rochester, MN 55901/USA

Consultant, National Cancer Institute; Lecturer, Department of Epidemiology and Public Health, Yale University School of Medicine; Clinical Assistant Professor, Department of Neurology, Georgetown University School of Medicine

Barbara W. Christine, Deceased; formerly Chief, Chronic Disease Control Section, Connecticut State Department of Health, Hartford, CT 06115/USA

Joseph F. Fraumeni, Jr., National Cancer Institute, National Institutes of Health, Bethesda, MD 20014/USA

Richard A. Greenberg, Department of Community Health, University of Louisville Medical School, Louisville, KY 40202/USA

Devera G. Schoenberg, Research Epidemiologist, Bethesda, MD 20014/USA

*Sponsored by the Swiss League against Cancer*

ISBN-13: 978-3-642-81069-5 e-ISBN-13: 978-3-642-81067-1
DOI: 10.1007/978-3-642-81067-1

Library of Congress Cataloguing in Publication Data. Schoenberg, Bruce S. (1942-
Multiple primary malignant neoplasms. Recent results in cancer research ; 58)
Bibliography: p. Includes index. 1. Multiple tumors. 2. Tumors--Reporting--Connecticut. 3. Cancer--Connecticut. I. Title. II. Series.
[DNLM: 1. Neoplasms--Occurrence--Connecticut. 2. Registries.
WI RE106P v. 58 / QZ200 S365m] RC261.R35 vol. 58 [RC262]
616.9'94'008s [616.9'94] 76-46556



Softcover reprint of the hardcover 1st edition 1977



2125/3140 — 543210

Dedicated to the memory of

| | |
|---|---|
| Charles Schoenberg | Louis Brodsky |
| Joseph Lieberman | Oliver Ross |
| Henry Eisenberg | Barbara Christine |

and the all too many who annually
succumb to cancer

The authors gratefully acknowledge the technical assistance of J. MICHAEL STUMP and NORMAN OSLIK in the intricate computer programming required for the analysis of the large volume of data presented in this monograph.

# Preface

When asked why he robbed banks, an astute and successful criminal is said to have replied "Because that's where the money is kept."

Why study patients with multiple primary cancers? The answer follows the same practical approach. Because the intensive investigation of such patients is very likely to yield data useful to both the clinical and research oncologist.

Studies of this problem provide an immediate return for the clinician responsible for the care of cancer patients. With improved forms of therapy, these individuals are enjoying longer periods of survival. One important factor in maintaining increased survival is the early detection and treatment of new primary tumors which may develop. Analyses of multiple primary malignancies serve as a guide to the probable anatomic location of a subsequent primary and help define characteristics of the individual at high risk for multiple primary cancer. But just as treatment may improve the life of the cancer patient, it may also increase the risk of a subsequent malignancy. Studies of multiple primaries provide an efficient means for quantifying potentially harmful effects of current therapeutic modalities.

The present study allows one to compare the observed and expected number of subsequent primary cancers. Tumors which occur together more often than expected may reflect a common etiology. Patients with more than one malignant neoplasm deserve careful study, as this occurrence may derive from an unusually high exposure to carcinogenic factors or unusually high susceptibility to such factors. The results of this study should mirror the findings of genetic, clinical, and laboratory endeavors in research oncology.

The tabulations presented in this monograph represent the *first and only* currently available systematic review of the multiple primary cancer experience of a large-scale, population-based tumor registry. Both the incidence rates used to calculate the expected numbers of subsequent cancers and the cohort of individuals under observation with a first primary cancer are derived from the same population. The Connecticut Registry has served as a high-quality data resource for over thirty years and is regarded as a model for cancer registration systems throughout the United States and abroad.

To carry out this investigation, the routine data collection and editing methods of the registry were supplemented by special efforts. This required a considerable investment of time and money and necessitated limiting the study to the period 1935—1964. Wherever possible, in order to reduce the chance of error, computer-generated tables were prepared in a format suitable for offset printing. Each chapter was written as a discrete unit, and although this procedure resulted in some duplication, the reader interested in particular forms of cancer can focus his attention on specific sections of the text without the need to scan the entire book. The interpretations in each chapter represent one opinion. In all cases, the results underlying these interpretations are provided. The reader is encouraged to form his own conclusions, based on these tabulations. Chapter 5 which discusses sources of bias in these analyses should be reviewed by anyone using these data. Finally, results of this investigation should not be interpreted as providing definitive answers, but rather should be regarded as stimuli to more intensive clinical, pathologic, and laboratory investigations. Only if these stimuli evoke appropriate investigative responses will this effort be considered a success.

Rochester, Minnesota

BRUCE S. SCHOENBERG

# Contents

*Chapter 1.* Historical Background 1
Importance of Tumor Registries 3
Connecticut Experience 4

*Chapter 2.* Materials and Methods 15

*Chapter 3.* Simultaneously Diagnosed Multiple Primary Malignant Neoplasms 19

*Chapter 4.* Non-Simultaneously Diagnosed Multiple Primary Malignant Neoplasms: General Considerations 22

*Chapter 5.* Non-Simultaneously Diagnosed Multiple Primary Malignant Neoplasms: The Connecticut Results and an Explanation of the Tabulations 29

*Chapter 6.* Index Tumors of the Buccal Cavity and Pharynx 33

*Chapter 7.* Index Tumors of the Digestive System 47

*Chapter 8.* Index Tumors of the Respiratory System 69

*Chapter 9.* Index Tumors of the Breast and Reproductive Organs 80

*Chapter 10.* Index Tumors of the Urinary System 108

*Chapter 11.* Index Tumors of Lymphatic and Hematopoietic Tissues 116

*Chapter 12.* Index Tumors of Remaining and Ill-Defined Sites 123

*Chapter 13.* Summary, Applications of these Data, and Perspectives for the Future 141

*References* 147

*Additional References* 154

*Appendix* 155

*Epilogue* 164

*Subject Index* 169

# Chapter 1

# Historical Background

In 1802, as members of the Society for Investigating the Nature and Cure of Cancer, a group of eight physicians and surgeons formulated a list of 13 questions to serve as a basis of further inquiry into the nature of malignant neoplasms (SCHOENBERG, 1975). One of these 13 queries addressed the issue of whether "... the existence of cancer in one part afford(s) a presumption that there is a tendency to a similar morbid alteration in other parts of the animal system." Their question was followed by reference to several anecdotal accounts of cancer involving both the breast and uterus (MEDICAL COMMITTEE OF THE SOCIETY FOR INVESTIGATING THE NATURE AND CURE OF CANCER, 1806).

John PEARSON, a surgical member of the Society had, some 9 years earlier, published a case report of cancer involving one breast, then the second breast, and finally the uterus (PEARSON, 1973). Such descriptions, although unusual, began to appear in the medical literature of the nineteenth century. There was still considerable confusion as to whether such cases represented examples of widespread metastases or rather instances of primary independent neoplasms.

BILLROTH, the first individual to establish a set of rigid criteria useful in defining the phenomenon of multiple primary neoplasms, provided a firm scientific basis for further descriptive studies. He wrote: "1) Each tumor must have an independent histologic appearance; 2) the tumor must arise in different situations; (and) 3) each tumor must produce its own metastases" (HANLON, 1931). These criteria were extremely restrictive and consequently were largely ignored by most medical writers. GOETZE in 1913 proposed a minor modification of these rules: "1) The macroscopic and microscopic appearance of the tumor must be that of the usual carcinomas of the organs involved; 2) the exclusion of metastases must be certain; (and) 3) diagnosis may be confirmed by the character of the metastases in each case" (HANLON, 1931).

In 1932, WARREN and GATES offered a set of definitions of multiple primary malignancies that have been widely adopted by other authors with little or no change. They wrote: "Each of the tumors must present a definite picture of malignancy, each must be distinct, and the probability of one being a metastasis of the other must be excluded." Four years later, BURKE (1936) adopted these same criteria. As an addendum to these rules, several authors have remarked on the necessity to exclude tumors with a known tendency to multicentric origin (AUSTIN, 1938; TULLIS, 1942). Despite the considerable effort that has been devoted to establishing such rigid criteria, some authors never specifically state the rules, if any, by which they decide whether a given cancerous lesion is indeed a second primary malignancy.

The early case reports were followed by series of cases based on the experience of individual surgeons, pathologists, or medical institutions.

While providing valuable clinical or pathologic descriptions, these data did not necessarily reflect an accurate picture of the occurrence of multiple primary cancer in a well-defined population. In order to generalize from the results of any such study, one must know the characteristics of the population yielding the specific statistics. It should also be emphasized that several case reports of two or more neoplasms occurring within the same individual do not constitute proof of a significant biologic association. The two tumors must be shown to occur together more frequently than might be expected on the basis of chance. Despite these problems, early investigations of multiple primary malignancies were useful in defining and documenting the phenomenon.

Finally, a number of case-control comparisons were carried out. Such investigations were based on the assumption that the cases under consideration were representative of all such cases, and that the controls were representative of the general population. Unfortunately, the validity of this assumption was unknown. In many instances, authors attempted to use rough estimates of cancer incidence in the general population as the comparison against which to judge data concerning multiple primary malignancies. The problem of developing suitable statistical methods became critical, for it was necessary to predict whether the occurrence of multiple primary neoplasms together in the same individual was simply the result of chance. At first, many authors merely gave their opinion on the matter, not relying on any accepted tests of statistical significance. In 1938, after being challenged on the validity of his statistical methods, AUSTIN replied: "Perhaps I overstated the case; a number of articles have attempted statistical analysis, comparing the population and cancer incidence, and multiple cancers seem to occur more often than chance would indicate. It is probable that this is significant, although I do not think it has been mathematically proved" (AUSTIN, 1938).

In 1934, BUGHER derived an equation for the probability of death from cancer during a given age span with a coincidental second malignancy. In the development of his analytic method he assumed "... that the mortality function may be used as a morbidity function without great error ... (and that) the error introduced by such an assumption is probably no greater than the intrinsic inaccuracy of the mortality data."

PELLER (1941) reasoned that since fewer than 20% of people over age 40 develop cancer, for about four-fifths of the population over age 40, the cancer risk is practically zero. He therefore believed that cancer susceptibility for the remaining one-fifth of the population in this age group is at least five times that indicated by data derived from the average population. Using this inflated rate for "cancer susceptibles," he concluded that a first skin cancer protected against the development of a possible new internal malignancy. Unfortunately, PELLER was unable to identify the "susceptible" fraction of the population. As noted by EPSTEIN (1954), PELLER could not "... state with certainty that a larger percentage would not develop cancer if they did not die of other causes."

In order to determine the number of observed and expected second primary cancers, LOMBARD et al. (1946) obtained expected values "... by multiplying person-years (of observation) by the age-sex-site specific incidence rate and reduced (these figures) when necessary by (appropriate) correction factors...." WATSON in 1953 used similar techniques.

Despite these elaborate methods and the large volume of data collected, studies were still inadequate in many respects. In 1961, MOERTEL et al. criticized the state of analyses of this subject up to that time. They wrote: "On the whole, the literature concerning this subject leaves the impression that the incidence of a second cancer of a different organ or tissue in patients whose first lesion has been treated successfully is probably equal to, and perhaps exceeds, that in the general population. However, convincing statistical evidence is still lacking, and because the establishment of an entirely adequate control group seems impossible at this time, no attempt at this type of analysis will be made in the present study."

## IMPORTANCE OF TUMOR REGISTRIES

The formation of tumor registries and the resulting implementation of efficient follow-up procedures greatly aided in identifying a sufficient number of individuals with multiple primary malignancies and greatly facilitated case-control studies of this phenomenon. A number of reports have been published based on the multiple primary cancer experience of the Memorial Hospital for Cancer and Allied Diseases in New York (ROBBINS and BERG, 1964; BERG, 1967, BERG et al., 1968; SCHOTTENFELD et al., 1969; BERG et al., 1970; SCHOTTENFELD and BERG, 1971; SCHOTTENFELD et al., 1974), and Charity Hospital in New Orleans (NEWELL et al., 1974a; NEWELL et al., 1974b; NEWELL et al., 1974c; NEWELL et al., 1975). Unfortunately, the underlying population from which these hospitals draw patients is not well-defined. This leads to difficulties in choosing an adequate control population with which to compare the results of the tumor registry tabulations.

The most sophisticated studies of multiple primaries have been based on data from well-defined population groups. A population-based tumor registry is ideal for such an analysis, particularly if it has a large, well-defined group under observation for a period of 10 or more years. The optimal methodology for this type of investigation is one which makes it possible to compare <u>the observed and the expected</u> number of subsequent primary malignancies. This is most conveniently done through a person-years approach. Such a procedure adjusts for the age and sex distribution as well as for the survival experience of patients with a first primary cancer. Details of this method and the rationale for its use are described in Chapter 2. It is best if the incidence rates used in this procedure are derived from the same population yielding the first primary malignancies. A population-based tumor registry fulfills this condition. Otherwise, differences between the observed and expected number of subsequent primaries might be attributable to differences in the characteristics between the population yielding the incidence rates and the population to which the rates are applied.

Such a person-years approach makes it possible to determine whether an individual with a malignancy in a particular organ or tissue has an increased, decreased, or unchanged risk of developing a later primary malignancy in the same or another organ or tissue. If the patient with one cancer had a decreased chance of developing a new malignancy, it may be that the presence of the first tumor in some way protected the individual; studies of the mechanism of such protection might be useful. If, on the other hand, one cancer placed the patient at higher risk for a subsequent primary malignancy, it may be that the same oncogenic factors are operating in the pathogenesis of both neoplasms. Such analyses are useful in identifying the high-risk cancer patient. It is these individuals who deserve further study with respect to possible etiologic factors.

## CONNECTICUT EXPERIENCE

Using the data resources of one such population-based tumor registry, GREENBERG (1959b) and BAILAR (1963) accumulated experience in terms of person-years of observation and used incidence rates from the same population yielding the first primary cancers. They now had an adequate control - made possible by the unique capabilities of the Connecticut Tumor Registry.

The Connecticut Tumor Registry, begun in 1941, maintains records on all Connecticut patients with a diagnosis of malignant neoplasm admitted to a hospital in the state or who have such a diagnosis on their death certificate. In addition, the registry routinely receives reports on Connecticut residents with a diagnosis of cancer seen at major referral centers in neighboring states. Data were also obtained retrospectively through 1935. An attempt is made to follow all patients from diagnosis to death, and it is estimated that fewer than 5% of the cases are lost to follow-up (GREENBERG, 1959b). In certain instances (e.g., intracranial tumors), benign neoplasms are also reportable to the registry. Information received from hospitals, physicians, and death certificates are coded according to a uniform format (END RESULTS SECTION, NATIONAL CANCER INSTITUTE, 1967), and the coded tabulations are placed on magnetic tape. The Connecticut Tumor Registry offers many advantages because the incidence rates used to calculate expected multiple primary cancers are obtained from the same population yielding the first primary cancers. The registry also has nearly complete reporting and a sufficiently large experience to allow comparisons to be made on an individual primary-site basis. Detailed descriptions concerning the operation of the registry have been reported (GREENBERG, 1959a; CONNELLY et al., 1968).

GREENBERG analyzed the multiple primary experience of the Connecticut Tumor Registry from 1935 through 1954. To minimize the possibility of mistaking metastatic disease for a new independent malignancy, his criteria were quite restrictive: 1) the cancer must have been specified as a second primary cancer by the reporting hospital; 2) the cancer must have been in a different anatomic site group from that in which the first primary cancer was located; and 3) an interval of 5 years must have elapsed between the diagnosis of the first primary cancer and the subsequent diagnosis of the second primary cancer. The data were analyzed in broad site groupings by using a person-years approach. He found an increased risk of cancers of the digestive system and genital organs in female breast cancer patients, and an excess of second primary cancers of the digestive system in patients with gynecologic malignancies (GREENBERG, 1959b).

BAILAR also used Connecticut Tumor Registry data to study the incidence of non-uterine tumors among uterine cancer patients. His statistical methods were similar to GREENBERG's. He restricted his definition of second primary cancers to those: 1) occurring outside the uterus, and 2) confirmed as "new and independent neoplasms" by microscopic confirmation (BAILAR, 1963).

Using GREENBERG's criteria, the findings of his previous study were reconfirmed, updated, and better defined by site within the digestive and genital systems by SCHOENBERG et al. (1969). For the first time the analysis was carried out using a digital computer. The Connecticut Tumor Registry was also used as a data resource for other investigations of the multiple primary cancer experience of patients with index tumors of the colon and rectum (SCHOENBERG and CHRISTINE, 1974), nervous system (SCHOENBERG et al., 1975), and female genital organs (SCHOENBERG and CHRISTINE, submitted for publication).

In each of these studies the excess risk of subsequent primary cancers was characterized by site, sex, and time interval following the first primary cancer. In these last three investigations, the only criterion for later primary cancer was that it be reported as such by the physician or hospital supplying the information. In all reports using Connecticut Tumor Registry material, skin cancers (other than malignant melanoma) are excluded from the tabulations. Skin cancers are often treated on an outpatient basis and consequently the tumor may not be reported to the registry.

A summary of the major papers concerning multiple primary cancers is given in Table 1. Although individual case reports and case series appear in the early portion of the table, they have generally been excluded in the review of more recent publications based on case-control comparisons. The table shows the frequency or number of multiple primary malignant tumors found by each author, together with his conclusions as to whether this occurrence is more or less frequent than expected, or whether it represents a chance phenomenon. These studies should be compared with caution. One must consider not only how many individuals were included, but also how long these individuals survived, i.e., how long they were exposed to the risk of getting a later primary cancer. The frequencies of subsequent primary cancer quoted from the various papers are not standardized for the survival of each population examined. Many of the reports listed in the table involved autopsy series in which nonsymptomatic cancers were more likely to be discovered than in clinical series. Some of these studies dealt with cancer of a particular organ or tissue, some involved both synchronous (with the multiple primary cancers appearing or being diagnosed simultaneously) and metachronous (with the multiple primary cancers appearing or being diagnosed at different times) tumors, and others restricted themselves to one type or the other. Finally, the various authors used different criteria in defining multiple primary cancer and different statistical methods in analyzing their results.

Table 1. Summary of the literature dealing with multiple primary cancers

| Author | Year of publication | Total cancer patients | Cases of multiple malignant tumors No. | Cases of multiple malignant tumors % of cancer cases | Conclusions* | Comments |
|---|---|---|---|---|---|---|
| WELLS | 1901 | -- | 3 | -- | 2 | Report of one case occurring in a dog and two cases quoted from literature |
| WOOLLEY | 1903 | -- | 37[A] | -- | 1 | Included skin cancers. A: Benign tumors also reported in this paper are not included in this figure |
| MAJOR | 1918 | -- | 628 | -- | 1 or 2 (?) | Included skin cancer, with cases from literature and one case reported by author |
| KILGORE | 1921 | 1,100 | 37 | 3.4 | 1 | Breast was only site considered |
| FRIED | 1928 | -- | -- | 0.1 (Estimate) | 3 | Report of two cases with an estimate of frequency of occurrence of multiple primary cancer |
| ORR | 1930 | 1,046 | 8 | 0.8 | 2 | Autopsy series |
| HANLON | 1931 | 710 | 18 | 2.5 | 2 | Autopsy series |
| WARREN and GATES | 1932 | 1,078 | 40 | 3.7 | 1 | Autopsy series. Figures quoted are from authors' own series. They also report statistics from other series |
| HURT and BRODERS | 1933 | 2,124 | 71 | 3.3 | 0 | Confirmation by microscopic diagnosis. Series included skin cancers |
| LUND | 1933 | 1,548 | 94 | 6.0 | 1 | Cancer of buccal mucosa |
| BUGHER | 1934 | 983 | 30 | 3.1 | 1 or 2[B] | Autopsy series. B: Depending on type of analysis |
| SCHREINER and WEHR | 1934 | 11,212 | 307 | 2.7 | 0 | Included skin cancer |
| BURKE | 1936 | 583 | 46 | 7.8 | 1 | Autopsy series. Excluded lymphomas and leukemias |
| AUSTIN | 1938 | 887 | 24 | 2.7 | 1 | Autopsy series |

Table 1. (continued)

| | | | | | | |
|---|---|---|---|---|---|---|
| KIRSHBAUM and SHIVELY | 1938 | 1,411 | 25 | 1.2 | 1 (?) | Autopsy series |
| STALKER, PHILLIPS, and PEMBERTON | 1939 | 2,500 | 113 | 4.5 | 1 | Mostly skin cancer |
| WARREN and GATES | 1940 | 1,149 | 237 | 20.6 | 1 | First primary cancers involved skin |
| PELLER | 1941 | 5,876 | 270 | 4.6 | 3[C] | Skin cancers were included. Of the base population, 2,146 were observed until death and 905 had an autopsy. C: See text for discussion of calculation on which conclusion was based |
| COOPER | 1942 | 1,790 | 106 | 5.9 | 0 | Skin cancer cases |
| PHILLIPS | 1942 | 1,400 | 226 | 16.0 | 0 | Confirmed by microscopic diagnosis. This series involved cancer of skin |
| TULLIS | 1942 | 1,044 | 21 | 2.0 | 1 | Confirmed by microscopic diagnosis. Autopsy series. Excluded lymphoma, leukemia, and tumors of multicentric origin |
| HELLENDALL | 1943 | 685 | 30 | 4.3 | 1 | Autopsy series |
| LOMBARD and WARREN | 1943 | 1,990 | 117 | 5.9 | 1 | Much skin cancer included in this study |
| SLAUGHTER | 1944 | -- | 1,868 | -- | 1 | Review of literature with addition of 40 new cases. No figures as to base cancer population are available. Cancer of the skin is included in this series |
| WARREN and EHRENREICH | 1944 | 2,829 | 194 | 6.8 | 1 | This series is a continuation of 1,078 cases reported in 1932 by WARREN and GATES. Autopsy study. Used criteria of WARREN and GATES |
| LOMBARD, LEVIN, and WARREN | 1946 | 2,981 | 309 | 10.3 | 1[D] | These figures are for people who had died by the conclusion of the study. D: This conclusion pertains to skin cancer followed by a second skin cancer and males with lip cancer followed by multiple skin cancer |

Table 1. (continued)

| Author | Year of publication | Total cancer patients | Cases of multiple malignant tumors No. | % of cancer cases | Conclusions* | Comments |
|---|---|---|---|---|---|---|
| MIDER | 1946 | 726 | 21 | 3.0 | 1[E] | Only colon cancer as first primary. E: Author concluded that patients with cancer in large intestine and breast have a predisposition to new cancers in these same organs |
| MUSTAKALLIO | 1946 | 1,068 | 119 | 18.6 | 1[F] | Only considered first primary cancers of skin. F: Predisposition in general to other cancer, especially skin cancer |
| WATSON | 1953 | 16,626 | 1,171 | 7.0 | 2 | Clinical series. Mostly skin cancer |
| EPSTEIN | 1954 | 3,006[G]<br>879[H] | 180[G]<br>51[H] | 5.9[G]<br>5.8[H] | 2 | G: First primary malignant cutaneous neoplasm followed by a malignant neoplasm not affecting skin--data from California Tumor Registry. H: Same type of cancers as noted previously--data from Highland-Alameda County Hospital |
| FRIED | 1958 | 1,514 | 24 | 1.6 | 0 | Autopsy series |
| MALMIO | 1959 | 27,712 | 650 | 2.3 | 0 | Of the cases, 18.3% did not have a pathoanatomical diagnosis. Skin cancers are included in this study |
| MACDONALD | 1960 | 9,723<br>6,538[I] | 1,010<br>579[I] | 10.7<br>8.9[I] | 0 | Skin cancers included. Diagnoses were confirmed by a pathologist except for multiple skin cancer. I: Excluding skin cancer of areas of skin exposed to sunlight |
| MOERTEL, DOCKERTY, and BAGGENSTOSS | 1961 | 37,580 | 1,909<br>1,049[J] | 5.1<br>2.8[J] | 0 | J: In different tissues. Used criteria of WARREN and GATES. Authors believe that quoted incidence rate is less than actual incidence rate |
| BAILAR | 1963 | 5,366 | 199 | 3.7 | 1[K] | Used criteria of WARREN and GATES. First cancer in this series was always in uterine |

Table 1. (continued)

| | | | | | | |
|---|---|---|---|---|---|---|
| | | | | | | cervix or corpus. K: For breast cancer following adenocarcinoma of uterine corpus, and urinary bladder tumors following cervical cancer |
| GREENBERG | 1959 | 60,911 | $260^{L}$ | 0.5 | $1^{M}$ | L: See text for criteria. M: For breast cancer followed by cancer of digestive system, peritoneum, or genital organs; and for cancer of genital organs followed by cancer of digestive system or peritoneum--only for cancers in females |
| PICKREN | 1963 | 2,094<br>2,094 | 232<br>$158^{N}$ | 11.1 | 0 | Autopsy series. N: "Clinically" diagnosed. Used criteria of WARREN and GATES. Excluded any case involving skin alone |
| THOMA | 1964 | 2,346 | 99 | 4.2 | 0 | Autopsy series. Used criteria of WARREN and GATES. All skin cancers except melanomas were excluded |
| EINHORN and JAKOBSSON | 1964 | 1,681 | 226 | 13.5 | $1^{O}$<br>$2^{P}$ | Report of patients with carcinoma of lip as index tumor. O: Only holds true for younger age groups (25-50 yrs.). P: Only holds true for older age groups |
| POLK, SPRATT, and BUTCHER | 1965 | 2,157 | 158 | 7.3 | 1 | Study of frequency of multiple primary malignancies in patients with colorectal carcinoma as first primary neoplasm |
| FISHER and KETCHAM | 1966 | -- | 18 | -- | $2^{Q}$<br>$1^{R}$ | Presented 18 new cases of multiple primary cancer. Conclusion drawn from review of literature. Q: For unrelated organ and tissue systems. R: For related organ and tissue systems |
| SPRATT and HOAG | 1966 | 13,510 | 272 | 2.0 | 2 | No criteria given for second primary cancers. Clinical series |
| BERG | 1967 | 4,667 | 95 | 2.0 | $1^{S}$ | First primary cancers were leukemia, lymphosarcoma, Hodgkin's disease, and myeloma. S: For prostate, bladder, endometrial, breast, and skin cancers following first primary cancers noted above |

Table 1. (continued)

| Author | Year of publication | Total cancer patients | Cases of multiple malignant tumors | | Conclusions* | Comments |
|---|---|---|---|---|---|---|
| | | | No. | % of cancer cases | | |
| BERG, HUTTER, and FOOTE | 1968 | 396 | 22 | 5.6 | 1[T] | T: Only considered first primary cancers in major salivary glands. The conclusion holds for second primary cancers in skin and breast |
| HAJDU and HAJDU | 1968 | 3,321 | 177 | 5.3 | 2 | Autopsy series. Used criteria of WARREN and GATES. Excluded known multicentric and paired organ tumors |
| SCHOTTENFELD, BERG, and VITSKY | 1969 | 6,447[U] | -- | -- | 1[V] | U: First primary cancers arising in stomach and lower digestive system. V: Conclusion holds for following site group combinations: 1) metachronous multiple primary cancers of large intestine; 2) cancer of cecum followed by cancers in large intestine or in other organs or tissues; 3) cancer of colon or rectum followed by cancers in other organs or tissues; 4) cancer of colon or rectum followed by cancer of breast; 5) cancer of rectum or rectosigmoid junction followed by cancer of urinary bladder; 6) cancer of colon followed by cancer of female genital organs, especially cancer of endometrium |
| BERGE, CEDERQVIST, and SCHÖNEBECK | 1969 | 4,895 | 572 | 11.7 | 0 | Autopsy series |
| SCHOENBERG, GREENBERG, and EISENBERG | 1969 | 11,212 | 290 | 2.6 | 1[W] 2[X] | Report of a population-based series. Only females with first primary cancers of the breast or genital organs were studied for the development of second primary cancer of the digestive system and genital organs. Multiple primary cancers occurring within 5 years of each other and/or within the same anatomic site group were excluded. W: Con- |

Table 1. (continued)

| | | | | | | |
|---|---|---|---|---|---|---|
| | | | | | | clusion holds true only for the following site groups in females: 1) first primary cancer of the breast followed by second primary cancer of the colon, uterine corpus, and ovary; 2) first primary cancer of the genital organs followed by second primary cancer of the colon; 3) first primary cancer of the uterus (corpus or cervix) followed by second primary cancer of the rectum. X: No association found for the other sites studied |
| BERG, SCHOTTENFELD, and RITTER | 1970 | 9,415 | 518 | 5.5 | 1[Y] | Study of incidence of multiple primaries in patients with index squamous cell carcinomas of the respiratory or upper digestive tracts. Y: Conclusion holds for all idex tumors studied except those arising in nasal cavities, paranasal sinuses, and nasopharynx |
| SCHOTTENFELD and BERG | 1971 | 11,556 | 537 | 4.6 | 1[Z] | Report of multiple primary neoplasms in females following breast and genital cancer. Z: Conclusion hold for following site group combinations: 1) index breast tumor followed by opposite breast and ovarian cancer; 2) index ovarian tumor followed by breast cancer; 3) endometrial cancer followed by breast cancer |
| NEWELL, KREMENTZ, ROBERTS, and KINNEAR | 1974 | 1,404 | 54 | 3.1 | 1[a]<br>2[b] | Report of multiple primary neoplasms in whites vs. blacks with Hodgkin's disease, leukemia, and myeloma. a: Only holds true for all index leukemia patients and for white males with index Hodgkin's disease. b: Holds true for all other index tumors studied |
| NEWELL, KREMENTZ, and ROBERTS | 1974 | 1,435 | 198 | 13.7 | 1[c]<br>2[d] | Report of multiple primary neoplasms in whites vs. blacks with initial cancer of the buccal cavity and pharynx. c: Conclusion holds for following: 1) white males with index tumors of lip and mouth; 2) black |

Table 1. (continued)

| Author | Year of publication | Total cancer patients | Cases of multiple malignant tumors: No. | Cases of multiple malignant tumors: % of cancer cases | Conclusions* | Comments |
|---|---|---|---|---|---|---|
| | | | | | | males with index tumors of salivary glands, mouth, and pharynx; 3) white females with index tumors of lip. d: Conclusion applies only to black females |
| NEWELL, RAWLINGS, KREMENTZ, and ROBERTS | 1974 | 8,773 | 493 | 5.6 | 1[e] | A study of multiple primary neoplasms in black females vs. white females with initial cancers of the breast and uterus. e: Only holds true for: 1) black females having index tumor of breast and cervix; 2) white females with index tumor of breast, cervix, and ovary |
| SCHOENBERG and CHRISTINE | 1974 | 20,812<br>121,460 | 949[f]<br>959[g] | 4.6<br>0.8 | 1[h] | Report of a population-based series. f: Metachronous malignancies in 20,812 patients with first primary colon or rectal cancer. g: Metachronous malignancies of the colon or rectum in 121,460 patients with a first primary cancer of any site. h: Conclusion only holds for following site groups: 1) colon cancer followed by cancer of the mouth, small intestine, rectum, uterine corpus, ovary, prostate, kidney and ureter, or bladder; 2) rectal cancer followed by cancer of the colon, ovary, or prostate; 3) colon cancer following malignancies of the rectum, uterine corpus, ovary, or soft tissue; 4) rectal cancer following malignant melanoma and cancer of the uterine cervix, uterine corpus, or thyroid gland |
| NEWELL, KREMENTZ, and ROBERTS | 1975 | 6,272 | 277 | 4.4 | 1[i]<br>2[j] | A study of multiple primary neoplasms in blacks vs. whites with initial cancer of the digestive organs. i: Holds true for following: 1) black and white females; 2) white |

Table 1. (continued)

| | | | | | | |
|---|---|---|---|---|---|---|
| | | | | | | males with initial cancer of stomach and ano-rectum. j: Applies to black males, only |
| SCHOENBERG, CHRISTINE, and WHISNANT | 1975 | -- | 135 | -- | 1[k] | Population-based series; only metachronous multiple primary cancers for which at least one of the primary sites was within the nervous system were studied. k: Only holds true for breast cancer and meningioma in females |
| SCHOENBERG and CHRISTINE | Submitted for publication | 17,405<br>60,056 | 716[m]<br>529[n] | 4.1<br>0.9 | 1[o] | Population-based series; only metachronous multiple primary cancers for which at least one of the primary sites was the female genital organs were studied. m: Metachronous malignancies in 17,405 female patients with first primary cancer of the genital organs. n: Metachronous malignancies of the genital organs in 60,056 female patients with a first primary cancer of any site. o: Conclusion only holds true for the following site groups: 1) cancer of the uterine cervix followed by cancer of unspecified female genital organs, rectum, bladder, pharynx, or lung and bronchus; 2) cancer of uterine corpus followed by cancer of unspecified female genital organs, breast, rectum, colon, or kidney and ureter; 3) ovarian cancer followed by cancer of the corpus uteri or colon; 4) cancer of unspecified female genital organs followed by esophageal cancer; 5) cancer of the uterine corpus following cancer of the breast or uterus; 6) cancer of the ovary following cancer of the small intestine, breast, rectum, or colon |

*Conclusion codes:
0: No conclusion is drawn concerning effect of one cancer on the probability of a second primary cancer.
1: Occurrence of one cancer increases probability that patient will develop a second primary cancer.
2: Occurrence of one cancer has no effect on probability that patient will develop a second primary cancer.
3: Occurrence of one cancer lessens probability that patient will develop a second primary cancer.

# Chapter 2

# Materials and Methods

The present study comprised 56,404 male and 65,056 female patients who were residents of Connecticut, were of known age, and had a first primary cancer diagnosed between 1935 and 1964, inclusive. These patients were admitted to a hospital in Connecticut or neighboring states or had a malignant neoplasm listed on their death certificates. All malignant neoplasms, with the exception of non-melanotic skin cancers, are coded, and the coded information is placed onto magnetic tape. The registry does not attempt to collect data on all skin cancer cases; skin cancers (other than malignant melanoma) may be treated on an outpatient basis and not be reported to the registry. Non-melanotic skin malignancies are therefore excluded from the present analysis.

The Connecticut Tumor Registry provides information on cancer cases over a period of more than 30 years for a well-defined geographic region with an average population of two million people. The population is fairly stable and there are good medical facilities available throughout the state.

Special care was taken to assure ascertainment of all cases of multiple primary cancer reported to the registry. Searches beyond the routine operation of the registry and review of information available on known or suspected cases of multiple primary malignant neoplasms were carried out. Selected cases were examined by a pathologist for histologic confirmation. These special reviews required considerable time and cost, and necessitated limiting the current analysis to cases diagnosed through 1964.

In order to compare the observed and expected numbers of subsequent primary cancers in the Connecticut population, the overall survival data for each patient with a first primary malignancy were converted to person-years of observation; that is, person-years of observation or exposure to the risk of developing a new primary cancer. The calculation is based on the assumption that the survival experience for five patients observed for 1 year is comparable to that for one person observed for 5 years, provided the risk of developing cancer remains constant over the 5-year period. Only patients with malignant neoplasms were considered. Person-years of observation were accumulated for each patient with a first primary cancer for each year of age, starting at the first diagnosis of a malignant neoplasm to death of the individual or the age at last follow-up. The cutoff date for follow-up was December 31, 1964.

These data were grouped separately according to the anatomic site of the first primary cancer, the patient's sex, and the survival time following the diagnosis. Three survival intervals were chosen: 1) between 1 and 12 months, inclusive, after diagnosis; 2) greater than 12 months and up to and including 60 months following diagnosis; and 3) more than

60 months after diagnosis of the first primary cancer. An example of the methodology involved in converting survival experience into person-years of observation is given as follows (Table 2):

Table 2. Example illustrating calculation of person-years of observation following first primary cancer of the breast

| Survival (mo.) | Age | Patient 1[a] P.Y.O.[c] | Patient 1[a] P.M.O.[d] | Patient 2[b] P.Y.O. | Patient 2[b] P.M.O. | Total experience for these two patients (yrs.) |
|---|---|---|---|---|---|---|
| | 0 | | | | | |
| | . | | | | | |
| | . | | | | | |
| | . | | | | | |
| | 45 | | 6 | | | 0.50 |
| 1-12 | 46 | | 6 | | | 0.50 |
| | 47 | | | | 6 | 0.50 |
| | 48 | | | | 6 | 0.50 |
| | . | | | | | |
| | . | | | | | |
| | . | | | | | |
| | 0 | | | | | |
| | . | | | | | |
| | . | | | | | |
| | . | | | | | |
| | 46 | | 6 | | | 0.50 |
| | 47 | 1 | | | | 1.00 |
| | 48 | 1 | | | 6 | 1.50 |
| 13-60 | 49 | 1 | | 1 | | 2.00 |
| | 50 | | 6 | 1 | | 1.50 |
| | 51 | | | 1 | | 1.00 |
| | 52 | | | | 6 | 0.50 |
| | . | | | | | |
| | . | | | | | |
| | . | | | | | |
| | 0 | | | | | |
| | . | | | | | |
| | . | | | | | |
| | . | | | | | |
| | 50 | | 6 | | | 0.50 |
| | 51 | 1 | | | | 1.00 |
| | 52 | 1 | | | 6 | 1.50 |
| | 53 | 1 | | 1 | | 2.00 |
| | 54 | 1 | | | 8 | 1.67 |
| > 60 | 55 | 1 | | | | 1.00 |
| | 56 | 1 | | | | 1.00 |
| | 57 | 1 | | | | 1.00 |
| | 58 | 1 | | | | 1.00 |
| | 59 | 1 | | | | 1.00 |
| | 60 | | 7 | | | 0.58 |
| | . | | | | | |
| | . | | | | | |
| | . | | | | | |

[a] Cancer of the breast diagnosed at age 45; patient survived 15 years, 1 month.
[b] Cancer of the breast diagnosed at age 47; patient survived 7 years, 2 months.
[c] P.Y.O. = person-years of observation.
[d] P.M.O. = person-months of observation.

If a woman with a recorded age of 45 years had a cancer of the breast and survived 15 years and 1 month, her age at diagnosis would average 45.5 years. During her first year of survival she would contribute 6 person-months of observation (P.M.O.) at age 45, and 6 P.M.O. at age 46. During the following 4 years, she would contribute 6 P.M.O. at age 46, 1 person-year of observation (P.Y.O.) each at ages 47, 48, and 49, and 6 P.M.O. at age 50. Finally, in the last survival interval, she would contribute 6 P.M.O. at age 50, 1 P.Y.O. at each age from 51 through 59, and 7 P.M.O. at age 60. If a second woman with a recorded age of 47 had cancer of the breast, and survived 7 years and 2 months at the date of last follow-up, then she would be, on the average, 47.5 years old at diagnosis. In the first year of survival she would contribute 6 P.M.O. at age 47, and 6 P.M.O. at age 48. In the following 4 years, she would contribute 6 P.M.O. at age 48, 1 P.Y.O. each at ages 49, 50, and 51, and 6 P.M.O. at age 52. In the final survival interval, she would contribute 6 P.M.O. at age 52, 1 P.Y.O. at age 53, and 8 P.M.O. at age 54. The person-months of observation can be converted into person-years of observation by dividing by 12. The total experience for these two patients is summarized in Table 2. What was done with these two hypothetical female patients with breast cancer can be done for all female breast cancer patients or for patients of a given sex with cancer of any anatomic site.

In this manner, the survival experience for all patients with a first primary cancer of a specific site was accumulated for each survival interval and age-sex group. The experience in each 5-year age group was totaled, giving 18 such categories for each sex and survival interval (ages 0-4, ..., 80-84, 85 and older). Age-, sex-, and site-specific incidence rates (SCHOENBERG, personal data; EISENBERG, 1966), were then applied to the appropriate person-years of observation to obtain the expected number of subsequent primary cancer for each age category, sex, site, and survival interval. Since the data covered by the monograph extend over 30 years, one must account for the possibility that over this period of time the risk of developing certain cancers has changed (e.g., the incidence rates for lung cancer have increased while those for stomach cancer have decreased). Person-years of observation were therefore collected separately by decade (1935-1944, 1945-1954, and 1955-1964) and corresponding decade-specific incidence rates were used. Thus, for each age-, sex-, site-, survival interval-, and decade-specific grouping, the following equation can be applied:

$$\text{P.Y.O.}_{\text{Site 1, Age, Sex, Survival Interval, Decade}} \times \text{I.R.}_{\text{Site 2, Age, Sex, Decade}} = \text{Exp.}_{\text{Site 1-Site 2, Age, Sex Survival Interval, Decade}}$$

where P.Y.O. refers to person-years of observation collected for patients with a first primary cancer at site 1 in a given age, sex, survival, and decade grouping who are exposed to the risk of developing a new primary cancer; I.R. represents the incidence rate, which is a measure of the probability of a new cancer developing at site 2 and is specific for the same age, sex, and decade as the P.Y.O.; and Exp. refers to the expected number of subsequent primary cancers at site 2 in individuals who already have a first primary cancer at site 1, and is specific for a given age, sex, survival interval, and decade. These results are then summed for all age and decade groupings to obtain the total number of expected subsequent primary cancers at each site for each sex and for each survival interval.

The criterion, in this monograph, for defining a subsequent primary cancer is that the cancer be designated as such by the reporting hospital or physician. The coded records of reported cases of subsequent primary cancers were selected and matched by case number with the first primary cancers to obtain the observed number of subsequent primary malignancies. These were then allotted to the appropriate site, sex, and survival interval combinations.

Since the probability of developing a subsequent primary cancer is small, the number of subsequent primary cancers can be expected to follow a Poisson distribution. The statistical significance of the results was tested with a table of significance factors for the ratio of a Poisson variable to its expectation (BAILAR and EDERER, 1964). When the number of observed cases was zero, statistical significance was tested against the values given in a table of confidence limits for the expectation of a Poisson variable (PEARSON and HARTLEY, 1958). The total Connecticut population is initially available for estimating the incidence rate of first primary cancer. Only those who have developed a first primary cancer are subsequently available for the estimation of the incidence of later primary cancer. The estimation of the incidence of first primary cancers therefore has negligible error in comparison with the estimation of the incidence of subsequent primary cancers, since the former estimate is based on a much larger sample size.

# Chapter 3

## Simultaneously Diagnosed Multiple Primary Malignant Neoplasms

Unfortunately, there are no practical statistical methods currently available for estimating the expected number of simultaneously diagnosed multiple primary malignant tumors. Because of this, it will not be possible to compare the observed experience with an expected experience. In the case of simultaneously diagnosed (synchronous) multiple primaries, we must restrict ourselves to a descriptive analysis of what was found. The Connecticut Tumor Registry defines synchronous multiple primaries as those diagnosed within the same month. The more malignant or life-threatening neoplasm is arbitrarily designated as the index or first primary cancer. If one of the pair, trio, etc. of simultaneously diagnosed primary malignancies cannot be so designated, the assignment to first or subsequent primary status is done at random.

Among the population of 121,460 patients with a first primary cancer, there were 1,265 instances in which another primary malignant tumor was diagnosed at the same time as the malignancy designated as the first primary. The occurrence of this phenomenon is analyzed by anatomic site in Table 3. In this table, however, no arbitrary distinction is made as to which of the tumors was the first primary cancer or the subsequent primary cancer. Thus, as noted in Table 3, there were two instances in which two cancers of the lip were diagnosed simultaneously; there was one instance of synchronously diagnosed tongue cancer and lip cancer, and so on.

One must exercise great caution in attempting to apply these figures to other populations. Although these data are derived from the well-defined Connecticut population, they are basically a function of the characteristics (age, sex, survival, ethnic background, social and environmental circumstances, etc.) of that population. Unless one is certain that a comparison group matches the Connecticut group in all such respects, generalization is fraught with danger.

Table 3. Analysis by anatomic site of instances in which another primary malignant tumor was diagnosed at the same time as a malignancy designated as a first primary cancer

| | LIP | TONGUE | SALIVARY GLAND | MOUTH | PHARYNX | ESOPHAGUS | STOMACH | SMALL INTESTINE | COLON | RECTUM | LIVER & BILIARY PASS | PANCREAS | NOSE AND SINUSES | LARYNX | LUNG AND BRONCHUS | OTHER RESP | BREAST | CERVIX UTERI | CORPUS UTERI | UTERUS, UNSPEC | OVARY | FEMALE GENITAL |
|---|---|---|---|---|---|---|---|---|---|---|---|---|---|---|---|---|---|---|---|---|---|---|
| LIP | 2 | | | | | | | | | | | | | | | | | | | | | |
| TONGUE | 1 | 0 | | | | | | | | | | | | | | | | | | | | |
| SALIVARY GLAND | 1 | 0 | 0 | | | | | | | | | | | | | | | | | | | |
| MOUTH | 1 | 5 | 0 | 3 | | | | | | | | | | | | | | | | | | |
| PHARYNX | 0 | 0 | 0 | 9 | 1 | | | | | | | | | | | | | | | | | |
| ESOPHAGUS | 1 | 5 | 0 | 3 | 2 | 0 | | | | | | | | | | | | | | | | |
| STOMACH | 0 | 0 | 0 | 0 | 1 | 7 | 1 | | | | | | | | | | | | | | | |
| SMALL INTESTINE | 0 | 0 | 0 | 0 | 0 | 0 | 1 | 0 | | | | | | | | | | | | | | |
| COLON | 1 | 0 | 1 | 1 | 2 | 1 | 24 | 9 | 90 | | | | | | | | | | | | | |
| RECTUM | 2 | 1 | 0 | 0 | 2 | 2 | 5 | 4 | 94 | 8 | | | | | | | | | | | | |
| LIVER & BILIARY PASS | 0 | 0 | 0 | 0 | 0 | 0 | 4 | 0 | 4 | 3 | 0 | | | | | | | | | | | |
| PANCREAS | 0 | 1 | 0 | 0 | 0 | 0 | 3 | 1 | 6 | 0 | 5 | 0 | | | | | | | | | | |
| NOSE AND SINUSES | 0 | 0 | 0 | 0 | 0 | 0 | 0 | 0 | 0 | 0 | 0 | 0 | 1 | | | | | | | | | |
| LARYNX | 1 | 1 | 0 | 3 | 3 | 3 | 1 | 0 | 3 | 1 | 1 | 0 | 0 | 0 | | | | | | | | |
| LUNG AND BRONCHUS | 1 | 1 | 0 | 3 | 2 | 3 | 5 | 0 | 5 | 9 | 4 | 1 | 0 | 4 | 5 | | | | | | | |
| OTHER RESP | 0 | 0 | 0 | 0 | 0 | 0 | 1 | 0 | 0 | 0 | 0 | 0 | 0 | 1 | 1 | 0 | | | | | | |
| BREAST | 0 | 0 | 3 | 1 | 1 | 1 | 12 | 0 | 31 | 16 | 1 | 2 | 1 | 0 | 0 | 0 | 101 | | | | | |
| CERVIX UTERI | 0 | 0 | 0 | 0 | 0 | 0 | 3 | 0 | 2 | 6 | 1 | 0 | 1 | 0 | 1 | 1 | 9 | 5 | | | | |
| CORPUS UTERI | 0 | 0 | 0 | 0 | 0 | 0 | 0 | 0 | 9 | 0 | 0 | 1 | 0 | 0 | 0 | 0 | 4 | 14 | 2 | | | |
| UTERUS, UNSPEC | 0 | 0 | 0 | 0 | 0 | 0 | 4 | 0 | 2 | 4 | 0 | 1 | 0 | 0 | 2 | 0 | 8 | 5 | 3 | 1 | | |

| | | | | | | | | | | | | | | | | | | | | | | OTHER | PROSTATE | TESTIS | OTHER MALE GENITAL | KIDNEY AND URETER | BLADDER | MELANOMA OF SKIN | EYE | NERVOUS SYSTEM | THYROID | BONE | SOFT TISSUE | LYMPHOMAS & MYELOMA | LEUKEMIAS | OTHER SITES |
|---|---|---|---|---|---|---|---|---|---|---|---|---|---|---|---|---|---|---|---|---|---|---|---|---|---|---|---|---|---|---|---|---|---|---|---|---|
| OVARY | 0 | 0 | 0 | 0 | 0 | 0 | 1 | 1 | 23 | 4 | 0 | 1 | 0 | 0 | 0 | 0 | 11 | 5 | 35 | 15 | 2 | | | | | | | | | | | | | | | |
| OTHER FEMALE GENITAL | 0 | 0 | 0 | 0 | 0 | 0 | 0 | 0 | 0 | 0 | 0 | 0 | 0 | 0 | 0 | 0 | 4 | 5 | 2 | 2 | 0 | 1 | | | | | | | | | | | | | | |
| PROSTATE | 3 | 1 | 1 | 3 | 1 | 3 | 15 | 1 | 31 | 18 | 3 | 7 | 0 | 2 | 24 | 0 | 1 | 0 | 0 | 0 | 0 | 0 | 3 | | | | | | | | | | | | | |
| TESTIS | 0 | 0 | 0 | 0 | 1 | 0 | 0 | 0 | 0 | 0 | 0 | 0 | 0 | 0 | 0 | 0 | 0 | 0 | 0 | 0 | 0 | 0 | 3 | 7 | | | | | | | | | | | | |
| OTHER MALE GENITAL | 0 | 0 | 0 | 1 | 0 | 0 | 1 | 0 | 0 | 0 | 0 | 0 | 0 | 0 | 0 | 0 | 0 | 0 | 0 | 0 | 0 | 0 | 0 | 0 | 0 | | | | | | | | | | | |
| KIDNEY AND URETER | 0 | 0 | 0 | 0 | 0 | 1 | 7 | 2 | 8 | 2 | 2 | 3 | 0 | 0 | 5 | 0 | 2 | 0 | 0 | 0 | 0 | 0 | 9 | 0 | 0 | 3 | | | | | | | | | | |
| BLADDER | 0 | 0 | 0 | 1 | 0 | 1 | 5 | 0 | 12 | 5 | 1 | 2 | 1 | 0 | 10 | 0 | 4 | 3 | 0 | 2 | 0 | 0 | 68 | 0 | 0 | 20 | 3 | | | | | | | | | |
| MELANOMA OF SKIN | 0 | 0 | 0 | 0 | 0 | 0 | 0 | 0 | 0 | 0 | 0 | 0 | 0 | 0 | 0 | 0 | 2 | 0 | 0 | 0 | 0 | 0 | 0 | 0 | 0 | 0 | 0 | 2 | | | | | | | | |
| EYE | 0 | 0 | 0 | 0 | 0 | 0 | 0 | 0 | 0 | 0 | 0 | 0 | 0 | 0 | 0 | 0 | 1 | 0 | 0 | 0 | 0 | 0 | 1 | 0 | 0 | 0 | 0 | 0 | 0 | | | | | | | |
| NERVOUS SYSTEM | 0 | 0 | 0 | 0 | 0 | 0 | 1 | 0 | 2 | 1 | 0 | 1 | 0 | 0 | 1 | 0 | 3 | 0 | 1 | 0 | 0 | 0 | 4 | 0 | 0 | 1 | 1 | 0 | 0 | 1 | | | | | | |
| THYROID | 0 | 0 | 0 | 0 | 0 | 1 | 4 | 0 | 0 | 0 | 1 | 0 | 0 | 0 | 0 | 0 | 0 | 0 | 0 | 0 | 0 | 0 | 1 | 0 | 0 | 0 | 1 | 0 | 0 | 1 | 0 | | | | | |
| BONE | 0 | 0 | 0 | 0 | 0 | 2 | 0 | 0 | 0 | 0 | 0 | 0 | 0 | 0 | 0 | 0 | 1 | 1 | 0 | 0 | 0 | 0 | 1 | 1 | 0 | 0 | 0 | 0 | 0 | 0 | 0 | 0 | | | | |
| SOFT TISSUE | 0 | 0 | 0 | 0 | 0 | 0 | 0 | 1 | 0 | 0 | 0 | 0 | 0 | 0 | 0 | 0 | 1 | 0 | 0 | 0 | 0 | 0 | 2 | 0 | 0 | 0 | 0 | 0 | 0 | 0 | 1 | 0 | 0 | | | |
| LYMPHOMAS & MYELOMA | 0 | 0 | 0 | 0 | 0 | 2 | 3 | 1 | 4 | 1 | 0 | 0 | 0 | 0 | 3 | 0 | 4 | 1 | 0 | 0 | 0 | 0 | 7 | 0 | 0 | 2 | 4 | 0 | 0 | 0 | 2 | 0 | 0 | 1 | | |
| LEUKEMIAS | 1 | 1 | 1 | 2 | 1 | 0 | 5 | 0 | 9 | 2 | 2 | 1 | 0 | 1 | 6 | 0 | 2 | 3 | 0 | 0 | 2 | 0 | 17 | 0 | 0 | 4 | 4 | 0 | 0 | 0 | 1 | 0 | 0 | 2 | 0 | |
| OTHER SITES | 0 | 0 | 0 | 0 | 0 | 1 | 3 | 0 | 1 | 8 | 1 | 2 | 0 | 1 | 2 | 0 | 7 | 3 | 0 | 0 | 0 | 1 | 6 | 0 | 0 | 1 | 8 | 0 | 1 | 3 | 1 | 1 | 0 | 0 | 4 | 0 |
| TOTAL | 15 | 16 | 6 | 30 | 17 | 28 | 109 | 20 | 336 | 88 | 22 | 22 | 4 | 9 | 60 | 1 | 165 | 45 | 43 | 20 | 4 | 2 | 122 | 8 | 0 | 31 | 21 | 2 | 1 | 5 | 5 | 1 | 0 | 3 | 4 | 0 |

# Chapter 4

# Non-Simultaneously Diagnosed Multiple Primary Malignant Neoplasms: General Considerations

In the case of non-simultaneously occurring multiple primary malignancies, available methods allow one to compare the observed and expected number of second primary cancers. Without the presence of an adequate control group, it is impossible to evaluate whether a reported association between two cancers simply represents a chance occurrence. It is imperative always to question whether a reported association is real or artifactual. In examining results of such investigations, one must constantly consider certain possibilities for bias. Problems inherent in the use of data from selected populations, establishing adequate statistical techniques, and utilizing a proper control population have already been discussed in Chapter 1.

Even when a person-years approach is applied to data from an unselected, well-defined population in order to minimize such error, other sources of bias remain. For example, metastatic disease may be mistaken for an independent primary malignancy. This problem of misclassification is likely to be greater when two tumors occur in close anatomic or temporal proximity. Therefore, histologic confirmation of the tumors as independent primary neoplasms is important. It may be that the group who already developed one cancer is more closely followed medically than the population who has not developed a malignancy, so that subsequent cancers are likely to be discovered more often and earlier in patients who have had a cancer. One must use clinical judgment in evaluating the results by considering the possible effects of treatment and problems in differential diagnosis. An example of an association due largely to artifact is the excess of prostatic cancer in males with first primary cancer of a variety of different sites. This relationship reflects: 1) the common diagnosis of occult primary prostatic cancer at autopsy, and 2) the fact that autopsies are more common in patients who have died of cancer than in the general population of deaths.

Finally, it should be emphasized that multiple comparisons have been made in the large-scale surveys of multiple primary malignancies and that some statistically significant results would be expected on the basis of chance. It therefore becomes imperative to distinguish biologic significance from statistical significance. Before accepting a statistically significant association as real, one must search for supporting evidence from other sources. It is more likely that a common etiologic mechanism is involved for site group combinations exhibiting a two-way association (cancer at site 2 occurs more frequently than expected in patients with cancer at site 1 and cancer at site 1 occurs more frequently than expected in patients with cancer at site 2) than for site-group pairs exhibiting a one-way association. Once possible sources of bias have been ruled out, one may then proceed with an exploration of the biological significance of the results.

A number of studies of multiple primary cancers have been based on an a priori hypothesis that patients with cancer at one site may be subject to an increased risk of cancer at the same or another site because of the presence of a particular etiologic factor (e.g., cigarette smoking, radiation, etc.). It is useful to summarize such investigations by categorization according to possible etiologic explanations (Table 4).

Table 4. Examples of site-group pairs with an excess of observed/expected subsequent primary malignancies

| Explanation of results | Anatomic sites or tumor types of multiple primary neoplasms |
|---|---|
| I. Common etiologic factors | |
| A. Same or paired organs | Colon ------------------ Colon<br>Breast ----------------- Breast |
| B. Chemical carcinogens | |
| 1. Tobacco | Upper respiratory and gastrointestinal tracts<br>Lung and bladder |
| 2. Mineral oil | Scrotum and lung |
| C. Endocrine and nutritional | Breast, uterine corpus, ovary, and colon<br>? Meningioma and breast |
| D. Genetic | Colon and uterine corpus<br>Retinoblastoma and lower extremity osteosarcoma<br>Multiple endocrine adenomatosis: tumors of anterior pituitary, parathyroid, pancreatic islet cells, and less frequently, neoplasms of thyroid, adrenal cortex, and carcinoid tumors of intestine and bronchus<br>Von Hippel-Lindau disease: hemangiomas of retina and cerebellum with excessive frequency of hypernephroma, pheochromocytoma, and ependymoma<br>Von Recklinghausen's disease: multiple neurofibromas, glioma, meningioma, acoustic neuroma, and pheochromocytoma<br>Pheochromocytoma, medullary thyroid carcinoma, multiple neuromas, and parathyroid tumors<br>Turcot's syndrome: polyposis of colon and brain tumors<br>Gardner's syndrome: polyposis of colon with osteomas, fibromas, lipomas, and epidermal cysts |
| II. Treatment | |
| A. Radiation | Rectal cancer following cancer of uterine corpus or cervix<br>Osteosarcoma, soft-tissue sarcoma, or skin cancer of orbit following retinoblastoma |
| B. Chemotherapy | Other neoplasms following Hodgkin's disease<br>Acute myeloblastic or acute myelomonoblastic leukemia following multiple myeloma<br>Squamous-cell carcinoma of urinary bladder following myeloma treated with cyclophosphamide |
| C. Surgery | Lymphangiosarcoma following breast cancer |
| III. Immune defects | Thymoma and other primary neoplasms<br>Chronic lymphatic leukemia and skin cancer |
| IV. Unknown etiologic significance | Breast and salivary gland |

Also included on the chart is the last grouping reflecting our current paucity of knowledge in the area of oncogenesis. Although associations of multiple primaries included in this last category may be expected because of the results of previous studies, the biologic mechanisms responsible for these associations remain obscure.

Again it is important to emphasize that one should always question whether a reported association is real or artifactual. Only after possible sources of bias have been ruled out, may one then proceed with an exploration of the biologic significance of the results.

The first category in Table 4 includes site-group combinations linked by possible common environmental or genetic factors. A number of studies demonstrate that colon cancer patients are at high risk for developing new, independent colon malignancies, and women with breast cancer are prone to cancer of the opposite breast (DENCKER et al., 1969; DEVITT et al., 1969; ROBBINS and BERG, 1964). This excess risk within the same organ or in paired organs might be explained by similar tissue being exposed to the same carcinogenic factors. The exact nature of the factors involved remains unknown, although hormonal, dietary, and genetic profiles of these patients are being evaluated.

Patients with cancer of the upper respiratory and gastrointestinal tracts have a tendency to develop a second neoplasm within this same anatomic location (BERG et al., 1970). Cigarette smoking, responsible for single tumors at these sites, also enhances the risk of multiple primary cancers of the mouth, pharynx, larynx, esophagus, and lung (HIGGINSON and MUIR, 1973; CASTIGLIANO, 1968; WYNDER et al., 1969; MOORE, 1971; SCHOTTENFELD et al., 1974). There is disagreement, however, as to whether cessation of smoking after the development of the first primary cancer lowers the risk of developing a second independent malignancy. Since lung cancer and bladder cancer are strongly correlated with cigarette consumption, one might expect to find a relationship between these tumors (LILIENFELD et al., 1956; DOLL and HILL, 1964). In the Connecticut tabulations (see Chapters 8 and 10), only a one-way association was found: an excess of second primary lung cancer among bladder cancer patients. The most likely explanation for the lack of a two-way association is that patients with lung cancer do not live long enough for bladder cancer to develop.

By studying a cohort of individuals who developed scrotal carcinoma attributed to industrial exposure to mineral oil, a group of investigators noted three patients with subsequent primary lung cancer. A follow-up survey of the survival experience of all scrotal cancer patients reported to a central tumor registry in the same geographic area revealed an excess of second primaries of the digestive and respiratory systems. Occupational exposure to mineral oil mist was suggested as the etiologic factor responsible for this association (EDITORIAL, 1970; HOLMES et al., 1970; KIPLING and WALDRON, 1976).

The group at high risk for one cancer may also be prone to other cancers because of common demographic factors (which may, of course, reflect common biologic factors). Investigations using registry data and employing the person-years approach adjust for age and sex in computing the number of expected later primary cancers. Therefore, these characteristics cannot be used to explain the reported associations.

Two registry studies document an association among cancers of the breast, uterine corpus, ovary, and colon in women (SCHOENBERG et al., 1969; SCHOTTENFELD et al., 1969). Numerous studies show that patients with breast cancer are more frequently unmarried, or if married, have lower pregnancy rates than comparable controls (HEIBERG and HEIBERG, 1940; HARNETT, 1948; GILLIAM, 1951; WYNDER et al., 1960; LILIENFELD, 1963). Similarly, endometrial cancer patients have a high frequency of infertility (SOMMERS et al., 1949; SPEERT, 1949; DOCKERTY et al., 1955; CORSCADEN, 1962). An investigation of the role of marital status in cancer mortality revealed that nuns have a higher risk of malignant neoplasms affecting the large intestine, breast, corpus uteri, and ovary than the general female population (FRAUMENI et al., 1969). Finally, a study of female patients with colon cancer reveals a higher proportion of infertility among these patients than among comparable controls (ACHESON et al., submitted for publication). Here we have a single factor, infertility or reduced fertility, which may be a function of some other factor(s), but which is associated with an increased risk of cancer of the female breast, colon, ovary, and corpus uteri.

In a paper correlating international death rates, WYNDER et al., (1967), compared mortality rates for cancer of the breast and colon in women for 21 countries, and found a positive correlation. They hypothesized that dietary habits may have a direct effect on increasing the risk of colon cancer in women, and an indirect effect, mediated through hormonal mechanisms, on increasing the risk of breast cancer.

The association between breast cancer and brain tumors was discovered in an analysis of Connecticut Tumor Registry data, and the relationship was limited to women with meningioma and breast cancer (SCHOENBERG, 1974; SCHOENBERG et al., 1975). Although yet to be substantiated by other investigations, this result raises interesting etiologic possibilities when considered in conjunction with other epidemiologic features of meningiomas. First, meningiomas are the only common intracranial neoplasm with a higher incidence in females (SCHOENBERG et al., 1976), and second, several authors have reported the abrupt appearance or enlargement of meningiomas during pregnancy (MICHELSEN and NEW, 1969). Thus, the association between breast cancer and meningioma may be related to hormonal factors.

Genetic investigations of cancer and studies of multiple primary malignancies complement one another. The same constellation of tumors occurring among members of the same family can also be found in a single individual. As noted by ANDERSON, hereditary cancers are often found 1) at several locations within one organ, 2) bilaterally in paired organs, or 3) at multiple sites within a specific tissue type, wherever this tissue exists in the body (ANDERSON, 1975).

The study by LYNCH et al. (1967) of six cancer-prone families revealed a frequency of multiple primary neoplasms above the figures from other papers dealing with large series of cancer patients. These families were distinguished primarily by the frequent occurrence of endometrial and colon carcinoma. Other investigators have reported similar families that point to genetic determinants, although environmental factors cannot be excluded with certainty (SAVAGE, 1956; HAUSER and WELLER, 1936).

A nationwide investigation of 1,623 children hospitalized with retinoblastoma, revealed 30 with a second primary cancer. In 11 such cases, the second tumor could not be attributed to radiotherapy for the retinoblastoma. Of the 11, 3 of the second primaries were osteosarcomas and 3 were brain tumors (JENSEN and MILLER, 1971). A second study dealing with 1,130 retinoblastoma patients reported the occurrence of 7 additional bone tumors in areas far removed from the radiation field. The results indicated an excess of second primary tumors, mainly osteosarcomas, in patients with bilateral disease. No such increase was found in patients with unilateral disease. Since a familial pattern is usually apparent in cases of bilateral retinoblastoma (and only in a small percentage of cases with unilateral tumors), these findings suggest a genetic mechanism is involved in the development of both the retinoblastoma and osteosarcoma (KITCHIN and ELLSWORTH, 1974).

Mendelian inheritance has been described in several syndromes involving specific histologic types of multiple primary neoplasms. Patients with multiple endocrine adenomatosis may develop independent neoplasms of the anterior pituitary, parathyroid, and pancreatic islet cells, and less frequently, carcinoids of the intestine and bronchus, and tumors of the thyroid and adrenal cortex (JOHNSON et al., 1967). Patients with von Hippel-Lindau disease have hemangiomas of the retina and cerebellum. These individuals are also at increased risk for developing hypernephroma, pheochromocytoma, and ependymoma (FRAUMENI, 1973). Von Recklinghausen's disease consists of multiple neurofibromas, and carries an increased risk of other neurogenic tumors: glioma, meningioma, acoustic neuroma, and pheochromocytoma (RUBINSTEIN, 1972). Pheochromocytoma and medullary thyroid carcinoma occur together in the same individual, or in different members of the same family, and are sometimes associated with neuromas and parathyroid tumors (SCHIMKE et al., 1966). The familial pattern seen in these syndromes is consistent with autosomal dominant inheritance.

Familial polyposis of the colon may be associated with brain tumors in the syndrome described by Turcot, or with osteosarcomas, fibromas, lipomas, and epidermal cysts in the constellation of Gardner's syndrome (TURCOT et al., 1959; BAUGHMAN et al., 1969; GARDNER and RICHARDS, 1953). Some doubt the existence of Turcot's syndrome as a distinct clinical entity since the brain tumors have been of diverse histologic types (TURCOT et al., 1959).

Only rarely are such familial syndromes detected by large-scale, site-specific analyses of tumor registry data. The association of tumors of one specific histologic type with tumors of another specific histologic type may be diluted by the large number of other histologic types included in the same site classification as the associated neoplasms. However, once a particular syndrome involving multiple primary neoplasms has been discovered, tumor registry data are very useful in identifying other examples of the syndrome.

One factor which may predispose to cancer is treatment (i.e., treatment for a first cancer may induce a second cancer). Tabulations from Connecticut indicate that patients with a first cancer of the uterine cervix or corpus are at increased risk for developing rectal carcinoma (SCHOENBERG and CHRISTINE, 1974). The carcinogenic effects of radiation, often used in treating genital cancer, should be considered as a possible cause of the later primary cancer (NOVAK and WOODRUFF, 1959; WILLSON et al., 1963). Thus, radiation for cancer of the uterine corpus or cervix may induce cancer in a nearby structure such as the rectum (SLAUGHTER and SOUTHWICK, 1957; SMITH, 1962; MACMAHON and ROWE, 1971; QIZILBASH, 1974). To explore this hypothesis more fully, the excess risk of rectal cancer following a uterine malignancy was analyzed by time interval between the first and subsequent cancers. The excess risk of rectal cancer was limited to the period 5 or more years following uterine cancer, which is consistent with possible radiation induction of the rectal carcinoma. The observed and expected number of later primary rectal cancers was calculated separately for those uterine cancer patients ever treated with radiation, and those never treated with radiation. The excess risk was limited to the group which had received radiation (SCHOENBERG and CHRISTINE, submitted for publication).

Another example of radiation-induced cancer is the excess occurrence of osteosarcomas, soft-tissue tumors, and skin cancers within the radiation field of children treated for retinoblastoma (JENSEN and MILLER, 1971). Other instances of cancer following medical irradiation have also been reported (HUTCHISON, 1976).

A study of subsequent primary malignancies in 425 patients treated for Hodgkin's disease revealed a relative risk for second primaries of 3.8 in those given intensive radiotherapy without intensive chemotherapy. Those treated with chemotherapy alone had a relative risk of 4.3, although because of the small number of cases, this was not statistically significant. In patients receiving intensive radiotherapy and intensive chemotherapy the relative risk increased to 29 (ARSENAU et al., 1972). These data suggest that chemotherapeutic agents and radiation may have multiplicative effects in oncogenesis. A possible carcinogenic role of chemotherapeutic agents has further support from a report concerning a total of 26 multiple myeloma patients who subsequently developed acute leukemia, primarily of the myeloblastic or myelomonoblastic types (KARCHMER et al., 1974). Each of these patients received some form of an alkylating agent. No such increase in leukemia among myeloma patients was noted before these antineoplastic drugs came into general use.

A recent report of the development of squamous cell carcinoma of the urinary bladder in four myeloma patients and one individual with Hodgkin's disease treated with oral cyclophosphamide over prolonged periods of time suggests a clinical carcinogenic effect for this antineoplastic drug (WALL and CLAUSEN, 1975).

The chemotherapeutic agents may produce this excess risk by any one of three possible means: 1) a direct carcinogenic effect (HARRIS, 1976), 2) a suppression of the immune system (PENN, 1976), or 3) an increase in survival, thereby providing a prolonged time interval for subsequent primary neoplasms to develop as a result of any oncogenic mechanism.

An analysis of the Connecticut multiple primary malignancy experience indicates an excess of soft-tissue tumors following breast cancer. These soft-tissue neoplasms were primarily lymphangiosarcomas of the upper extremity, a known sequela of radical mastectomy and resulting obstructive lymphedema (STEWART and TREVES, 1948).

Thus, various modalities employed in treating cancer may in themselves increase the patient's risk of developing a new primary neoplasm.

It has been shown that kidney transplant patients receiving immunosuppressive therapy have an elevated risk of cancer, particularly lymphoreticular neoplasms and skin cancer (PENN and STARZL, 1972). Moreover, patients with immunodeficiency syndromes have a high frequency of leukemia and lymphoreticular tumors (KERSEY et al., 1973). The question arises as to whether these patients have an intrinsic abnormality of their reticuloendothelial system which leads to malignant transformation, or whether the high occurrence of malignancies is the result of the immunosuppression. Observations such as these have prompted much interest in the occurrence of second primary cancers in patients with a first primary malignancy of organs involved in the immune response.

SOUADJIAN et al. (1968) discovered that 21% of 146 thymoma patients followed for 20 years developed a non-thymic malignancy. This was in excess of the risk of second primary neoplasms found among a group of parathyroid tumor patients serving as controls. Berg has reported an excess of subsequent skin cancer developing in patients with lymphoma and leukemia, particularly chronic lymphatic leukemia or chronic myelogenous leukemia (BERG, 1967). Using tabulations from the Charity Hospital Tumor Registry, NEWELL et al. (1974a) also found an excess of skin cancer among white patients with Hodgkin's disease or leukemia, but felt these observations might be due to artifacts of reporting. MORIARTY (1974) reported that patients with chronic lymphatic leukemia are prone to skin cancer, and suggested that the excess of skin cancer was the result of immunologic incompetence among these patients.

Multiple tumors in organs apparently unrelated functionally or anatomically are not readily explained, but may be valuable in providing clues to etiology. Such associations may allow us to relate a tumor whose epidemiologic pattern is unknown to one whose epidemiologic pattern has been well delineated. The relationship between cancer of the breast and salivary gland was discovered by BERG et al. (1968) and has been substantiated by data from the Connecticut Tumor Registry (Chapter 6). However, the etiology of this relationship remains obscure.

# Chapter 5

# Non-Simultaneously Diagnosed Multiple Primary Malignant Neoplasms: The Connecticut Results and an Explanation of the Tabulations

The remainder of the monograph will be devoted to the experience of the Connecticut Tumor Registry with regard to multiple primary malignancies not diagnosed at the same time. Throughout this volume, the word "cancer" is used in a broad sense to denote malignant neoplasms and includes both carcinomas and sarcomas. The word "tumor" is used to denote a neoplasm, and not simply a "swelling." Anatomic sites containing more than one organ or tissue are often designated by a virgule between the organs or tissues involved; e.g., kidney and ureter would be designated as kidney/ureter.

The data presented will consist largely of a series of tables comparing the observed and expected number of subsequent primary malignancies by primary anatomic site and sex. For those site groups showing a substantial discrepancy between the observed and expected numbers of subsequent primary cancers, the data are further analyzed by time interval between the neoplasms. The present chapter is designed to aid the reader in interpreting these tables.

There are 37 basic tables (36 dealing with major anatomic sites and an overall summary table) analyzing the material according to separate anatomic sites and sex. Each of these tables follows the same format. The following definitions are used throughout this series of tabulations:

First Primary Site snd Subsequent Primary Site. The anatomic location of the first primary cancer and the subsequent primary cancer, respectively. Each of these sites is precisely defined with reference to a standard system of nomenclature in the appendix to this volume.

Number of Persons. The number of individuals who had a first cancer in the given primary site and who were at risk for developing a second primary cancer.

Person-Years of Observation. Person-years at risk for developing a second primary cancer (number of persons at risk X number of years during which these individuals are at risk).

OBS. Observed number of subsequent primary malignancies.

EXP. Expected number of subsequent primary malignancies. A value of 0.0 in this column means the result is less than 0.005.

OBS/EXP. Ratio of observed-to-expected subsequent primary malignancies. A value of 0.0 means the result is less than 0.005. A single asterisk (*) next to the ratio means the result is statistically significant at the 5% level. In other words, the probability of obtaining by chance a ratio as far as or further from 1.00 than the quoted ratio is less than

5%. A double asterisk (**) next to the ratio means the result is statistically significant at the 1% level.

The tabulations in the remaining chapters were produced by computer, which carried out the analysis to many more significant digits than indicated in the tables. The figures in the tables represent these computations rounded to the nearest hundredth. Because of this, additions based on data appearing in the tables may differ sightly from the total, calculated on the basis of many more significant digits by the computer.

Throughout the tabulations, there are several examples of ratios of observed-to-expected subsequent primary cancers in which OBS/EXP = 0/0.0 = 0.0. Such ratios do not represent the division of zero by zero. In these instances, the value for "EXP" is in fact very small, and is rounded to "0.0" when printed. Thus, the ratio, OBS/EXP = 0/0.0 = 0.0, represents division of zero by a very small, non-zero number.

Each of these basic tables is followed by a series of smaller tables presenting more detailed results only for site groups in which the ratio of observed-to-expected departs significantly from 1.00. In this second group of tabulations, the data are analyzed separately by time interval between the two tumors. The terms used in the basic tables are again repeated in these tabulations and carry the same meaning, with the following additions and modifications:

Years < 1. Results for all subsequent primary cancers diagnosed between 1 and 12 months, inclusive, after diagnosis of the first primary. Malignancies discovered within the same month are considered to be simultaneously diagnosed.

Years 1-5. Results for all subsequent primary cancers diagnosed between 13 and 60 months, inclusive, after diagnosis of the first primary.

Years > 5. Results for all subsequent primary cancers diagnosed more than 60 months after diagnosis of the first primary.

Terms such as "Number of Persons," "Person-Yrs of Observation," "Obs," "Exp," "Obs/Exp" carry the same meaning as defined previously, but are specific for the given time interval between the diagnosis of the first and the subsequent primary tumor.

The column labelled "Total" reflects the overall experience without division by time period. If, for any group of multiple primaries, the ratio of observed-to-expected subsequent primary cancers differs significantly from 1.00 in any of the time intervals, in any of the sex-specific analyses, or for the total period, the results are shown in the smaller tables. Site groups for which the ratio of observed-to-expected subsequent primaries does not depart significantly from 1.00 do not appear in this second series of tables. The results analyzed by time interval are of particular value in highlighting when after the diagnosis of a first primary cancer, the patient is at a particularly high risk or a particularly low risk for developing a subsequent primary malignant neoplasm. These tabulations may also provide clues to the oncogenic process. For example, concentration of high risk in a certain period following the diagnosis of a first cancer may suggest a specific set of possible etiologic agents.

The general problems of bias and artifact inherent in all studies of multiple primary malignant neoplasms were discussed in detail in Chapter 4. It is also necessary to point out possible sources of bias present in the analysis of the Connecticut data. The problem of misclassifying metastases as primary neoplasms and vice versa is likely to be greatest when the two lesions occur in the same anatomic location or in close temporal proximity. Great caution must therefore be used in interpreting reported multiple primary tumors occurring in such circumstances.

The loss of patients to follow-up (estimated to be about 5% among Connecticut residents) leads to a reduction in person-years of observation and a slight underestimation of the expected number of second primary cancers. It is less likely that second primary cancer cases would be lost to follow-up as the patients would probably come to medical attention.

Cases reported by death certificate only are included in the calculation of incidence rates. Use of the age at death for the age at diagnosis tends to increase the incidence rates for older age groups.

It may be that the group who already developed one cancer is more closely followed medically than the population who has not developed a malignancy, so that subsequent cancers are likely to be discovered more often and earlier in patients who have had a cancer. The group with one cancer already diagnosed may be more health conscious, or may come from areas of the state with better medical diagnostic facilities than the population in general, so that any second cancer may be diagnosed earlier.

As with all other large-scale surveys of multiple primary malignancies, multiple comparisons have been made without a priori hypotheses. One may therefore expect some statistically significant results on the basis of chance.

In summary, the limitations of the material presented in this monograph include the following:

1) Subsequent primary cancers are defined solely as being specified as such by the reporting physician or hospital.

2) Multiple comparisons have been made so that some significant results would be expected on the basis of chance.

3) While some of the significant findings are the result of biologic factors, the reader is cautioned to consider problems in differential diagnosis as an explanation of the findings.

To aid the reader in evaluating the difficulties of distinguishing between primary neoplasms and metastases, the third series of tables for each major anatomic site provides figures on the number of first and second primary cancers which were histologically confirmed as distinct, independent neoplasms. Microscopic confirmation is an important and necessary adjunct in the recognition of independent primary tumors.

Tables pertaining to each of the individual 36 major anatomic sites are grouped together according to seven organ systems: 1) buccal cavity and pharynx; 2) digestive system; 3) respiratory system; 4) breast and reproductive organs; 5) urinary system; 6) lymphatic and hematopoietic tissues; and 7) remaining and ill-defined sites. A chapter of the monograph is devoted to each of these seven systems. Included in each is a list of common metastatic sites for tumors originating in that organ system. This list, together with the figures for microscopic confirmation, should provide a useful guide for evaluating the accuracy of the clinical diagnosis of multiple primaries.

Also included in each chapter is an outline of all significant findings. An arrow pointing in one direction between sites indicates that patients with cancer at one particular site are at increased risk for cancer at the second site (to which the arrow is pointing). A bidirectional arrow joining tumor sites indicates a two-way association. In this case, patients with cancer at either site are at increased risk for cancer at the other site. It would seem likely that a common etiologic agent is responsible for the pathogenesis of the two tumors.

Each chapter includes a consideration of sources of bias and artifactual associations applicable to that particular organ system under consideration and a discussion of the possible biologic significance of the findings with appropriate supporting evidence from other epidemiologic and laboratory investigations.

The classification of associations as being possibly artifactual or possibly real is based on the number of observed cases, whether the relationship is unidirectional or bidirectional, the degree of microscopic verification of the multiple primary cancers, the likelihood of mistaking metastatic disease for a new primary cancer and vice versa, corroboration of the association by other investigators, and the recognition of biological mechanisms responsible for the relationship. However, the reader is cautioned not to accept this categorization as dogma, but rather to evaluate the data on his own in the light of new findings.

The reader may have preferred a finer division by anatomic site than shown in the tables (e.g., a separate listing for adrenal gland, pituitary gland, etc.). More detailed analyses such as these were carried out, but they provided no new insights into the associations reported nor did they reveal new relationships. In the interest of brevity, these tabulations were not included in the monograph.

# Chapter 6

# Index Tumors of the Buccal Cavity and Pharynx

Population Studied. A total of 5,777 patients with a primary malignant tumor of the buccal cavity or pharynx were followed for the subsequent development of independent primary malignant neoplasms; 491 such subsequent neoplasms were discovered. 81.3% of the patients with cancer of the buccal cavity and pharynx were male. This cohort of individuals contributed approximately 24,130 person-years of observation.

Results. Detailed tabulations by site are presented in Tables 5-19. The reader is referred to Chapter 5 for a general explanation of the items in these tables.

Summary of Findings. Site-group pairs with a statistically significant excess of observed-over-expected subsequent primary cancers are categorized in Table 20 on the basis of possible relationships between the anatomic sites containing these cancers. In addition, possible artifactual relationships, based on a small number of cases and with no confirmation from other published reports, are emphasized.

Discussion. Before examining the results critically, one must decide whether the findings are real or due to artifact. To aid in this respect Table 21 presents the common metastatic sites for cancers arising within the buccal cavity and pharynx. One must examine this in conjunction with tabulations of the percentage of multiple primary tumors with histologic confirmation by site. These are only shown for sites with a significant excess of observed-over-expected second primary cancers.

The association of tumors noted in the first category is thought to be the result of artifact. When so many comparisons are made, some will show a statistically significant excess of observed-over-expected second primary cancers on the basis of chance. The site-group pairs shown in this category are not supported by the findings from other investigations. With the exception of the excess of prostatic cancer following cancer of the mouth, the other associations are based on fewer than three observed cases. The statistically significant relationship between cancer of the mouth and prostate is thought to be the result of a large number of prostatic cancers discovered at autopsy for patients dying with cancer of the mouth.

Findings classified in group II of Table 20 include malignant tumors involving organs belonging to the same system, or organs which are related structurally and functionally. A number of other large-scale studies have reported multiple primary malignant neoplasms arising multicentrically within the buccal cavity and pharynx, and have described the association between buccal cavity and pharyngeal cancers with malignancies of the respiratory system and upper digestive tract (MOERTEL, 1966; BERG et al., 1970; NEWELL et al., 1974b).

With such relationships one is tempted to hypothesize the presence of a common carcinogen coming into contact with tissues of the buccal cavity, pharynx, respiratory system, and upper digestive system. SCHOTTENFELD et al. (1974) studied the potential role of alcohol and tobacco use in the etiology of this constellation of multiple primaries. After collecting careful histories of smoking and alcohol consumption from a cohort of individuals with single primary cancer of either the oral cavity, pharynx, or larynx, they monitored the group for the development of subsequent primary cancer of the upper digestive system, larynx, or lung. Furthermore, they noted any changes in the smoking and drinking patterns of this cohort. The risk of developing a second cancer was increased significantly by intensive combined exposures to alcohol and tobacco before the symptomatic onset of the first cancer. Within the first 5 years after the onset of the first cancer, a change in smoking or drinking habits of the patients did not affect the risk of developing a second cancer. In any case, the investigation suggests an association between heavy consumption of alcohol and tobacco and multiple primary malignancies of the oral cavity, pharynx, respiratory system, and upper digestive system. Tobacco and alcohol have also been associated with single cancers developing at these same sites (WYNDER and BROSS, 1961; KELLER and TERRIS, 1965; SCHOENBERG et al., 1971; ROTHMAN, 1975; HAMMOND, 1975).

BERG et al. (1968) first reported that women with a malignant neoplasm of the salivary gland were at a significantly increased risk for developing breast cancer. Their study was based on an analysis of cases seen at the Memorial Hospital for Cancer and Allied Diseases. With regard to the Connecticut experience for patients having cancer of the salivary gland, although the excess risk of breast cancer is statistically significant for males, it is not so for females. For only two of the four patients with cancer of the salivary gland and breast were both neoplasms microscopically confirmed. However, as noted in Tables 21 and 93, the breast is not a common metastatic site for cancer of the salivary gland, and vice versa. It therefore appears unlikely that the histologically unverified neoplasms represent metastatic disease. In any case, if this association has some biologic basis, the underlying mechanism remains unknown. But even the statistical association has been challenged. Reported results from the California Tumor Registry (DUNN et al., 1972) find an excess risk of breast cancer among women with cancer of the salivary gland, but the excess is not statistically significant. Two studies, one using the Mayo Clinic data (MOERTEL and ELVEBACK, 1969) and one analyzing the experience of Charity Hospital in New Orleans (NEWELL et al., 1974b) failed to document any increased risk.

Table 5. Subsequent multiple primary malignancies in patients with an index malignant tumor of the lip

FIRST PRIMARY SITE - LIP

| SUBSEQUENT PRIMARY SITES | TOTAL<br>NUMBER OF PERSONS= 1389<br>PERSON-YRS OF OBSERVATION = 10339.1<br>OBS | <br><br><br>EXP | <br><br><br>OBS/EXP | MALES<br>NUMBER OF PERSONS= 1302<br>PERSON-YRS OF OBSERVATION = 9856.1<br>OBS | <br><br><br>EXP | <br><br><br>OBS/EXP | FEMALES<br>NUMBER OF PERSONS= 87<br>PERSON-YRS OF OBSERVATION = 483.0<br>OBS | <br><br><br>EXP | <br><br><br>OBS/EXP |
|---|---|---|---|---|---|---|---|---|---|
| LIP | 7 | 2.15 | 3.26* | 7 | 2.14 | 3.27* | 0 | 0.01 | 0.0 |
| TONGUE | 9 | 1.63 | 5.53** | 9 | 1.61 | 5.58** | 0 | 0.01 | 0.0 |
| SALIVARY GLAND | 2 | 0.40 | 5.05 | 2 | 0.38 | 5.24 | 0 | 0.01 | 0.0 |
| MOUTH | 7 | 2.12 | 3.30* | 7 | 2.09 | 3.34* | 0 | 0.03 | 0.0 |
| PHARYNX | 4 | 2.03 | 1.97 | 4 | 2.01 | 1.99 | 0 | 0.02 | 0.0 |
| ESOPHAGUS | 4 | 3.76 | 1.06 | 3 | 3.74 | 0.80 | 1 | 0.04 | 27.83 |
| STOMACH | 12 | 13.62 | 0.88 | 12 | 13.21 | 0.91 | 0 | 0.41 | 0.0 |
| SMALL INTESTINE | 1 | 0.43 | 2.33 | 1 | 0.41 | 2.45 | 0 | 0.02 | 0.0 |
| COLON | 21 | 15.53 | 1.35 | 20 | 14.77 | 1.35 | 1 | 0.76 | 1.32 |
| RECTUM | 12 | 9.96 | 1.20 | 11 | 9.65 | 1.14 | 1 | 0.31 | 3.19 |
| LIVER & BILIARY PASS | 2 | 2.97 | 0.67 | 2 | 2.79 | 0.72 | 0 | 0.18 | 0.0 |
| PANCREAS | 6 | 5.00 | 1.20 | 6 | 4.83 | 1.24 | 0 | 0.17 | 0.0 |
| NOSE AND SINUSES | 0 | 0.30 | 0.0 | 0 | 0.29 | 0.0 | 0 | 0.01 | 0.0 |
| LARYNX | 6 | 2.73 | 2.20 | 6 | 2.73 | 2.20 | 0 | 0.01 | 0.0 |
| LUNG AND BRONCHUS | 24 | 14.90 | 1.61* | 24 | 14.78 | 1.62* | 0 | 0.12 | 0.0 |
| OTHER RESP | 2 | 0.23 | 8.54* | 1 | 0.23 | 4.34 | 1 | 0.00 | 269.38** |
| BREAST | 1 | 1.40 | 0.72 | 0 | 0.30 | 0.0 | 1 | 1.10 | 0.91 |
| CERVIX UTERI | 0 | 0.22 | 0.0 | 0 | 0.0 | 0.0 | 0 | 0.22 | 0.0 |
| CORPUS UTERI | 0 | 0.20 | 0.0 | 0 | 0.0 | 0.0 | 0 | 0.20 | 0.0 |
| UTERUS,UNSPEC | 1 | 0.14 | 6.96 | 0 | 0.0 | 0.0 | 1 | 0.14 | 6.96 |
| OVARY | 0 | 0.20 | 0.0 | 0 | 0.0 | 0.0 | 0 | 0.20 | 0.0 |
| OTHER FEMALE GENITAL | 0 | 0.06 | 0.0 | 0 | 0.0 | 0.0 | 0 | 0.06 | 0.0 |
| PROSTATE | 29 | 24.61 | 1.14 | 28 | 24.61 | 1.14 | 0 | 0.0 | 0.0 |
| TESTIS | 1 | 0.24 | 4.24 | 1 | 0.24 | 4.24 | 0 | 0.0 | 0.0 |
| OTHER MALE GENITAL | 0 | 0.48 | 0.0 | 0 | 0.48 | 0.0 | 0 | 0.0 | 0.0 |
| KIDNEY AND URETER | 2 | 2.74 | 0.73 | 2 | 2.67 | 0.75 | 0 | 0.07 | 0.0 |
| BLADDER | 7 | 9.40 | 0.74 | 7 | 9.24 | 0.76 | 0 | 0.16 | 0.0 |
| MELANOMA OF SKIN | 2 | 0.71 | 2.81 | 2 | 0.68 | 2.95 | 0 | 0.03 | 0.0 |
| EYE | 0 | 0.23 | 0.0 | 0 | 0.22 | 0.0 | 0 | 0.01 | 0.0 |
| NERVOUS SYSTEM | 0 | 0.94 | 0.0 | 0 | 0.91 | 0.0 | 0 | 0.04 | 0.0 |
| THYROID | 1 | 0.37 | 2.72 | 1 | 0.33 | 3.01 | 0 | 0.04 | 0.0 |
| BONE | 0 | 0.35 | 0.0 | 0 | 0.33 | 0.0 | 0 | 0.01 | 0.0 |
| SOFT TISSUE | 0 | 0.77 | 0.0 | 0 | 0.74 | 0.0 | 0 | 0.02 | 0.0 |
| LYMPHOMAS & MYELOMA | 6 | 3.25 | 1.85 | 6 | 3.14 | 1.91 | 0 | 0.11 | 0.0 |
| LEUKEMIAS | 8 | 3.76 | 2.13 | 7 | 3.65 | 1.92 | 1 | 0.11 | 8.79 |
| OTHER SITES | 9 | 6.88 | 1.31 | 9 | 6.59 | 1.37 | 0 | 0.30 | 0.0 |
| TOTAL | 185 | 134.71 | 1.37** | 178 | 129.80 | 1.37** | 7 | 4.91 | 1.42 |

Table 6. Subsequent primary sites with excesses

FIRST PRIMARY SITE - LIP

| SUBSEQUENT PRIMARY SITES | TOTAL | | | YEARS < 1 | | | YEARS 1-5 | | | YEARS > 5 | | |
|---|---|---|---|---|---|---|---|---|---|---|---|---|
| | NUMBER OF PERSONS= 1389 PERSON-YRS OF OBSERVATION= 10339.1 | | | NUMBER OF PERSONS= 1389 PERSON-YRS OF OBSERVATION= 1321.7 | | | NUMBER OF PERSONS= 1247 PERSON-YRS OF OBSERVATION= 3863.0 | | | NUMBER OF PERSONS= 757 PERSON-YRS OF OBSERVATION= 5154.4 | | |
| | OBS | EXP | OBS/EXP | OBS | EXP | OBS/EXP | OBS | EXP | OBS/EXP | OBS | EXP | OBS/EXP |
| LIP | 7 | 2.15 | 3.26* | 1 | 0.27 | 3.72 | 5 | 0.74 | 6.73** | 1 | 1.14 | 0.88 |
| TONGUE | 9 | 1.63 | 5.53** | 0 | 0.19 | 0.0 | 3 | 0.57 | 5.28* | 6 | 0.87 | 6.88** |
| SALIVARY GLAND | 2 | 0.40 | 5.05 | 0 | 0.04 | 0.0 | 0 | 0.13 | 0.0 | 2 | 0.22 | 9.09* |
| MOUTH | 7 | 2.12 | 3.30* | 1 | 0.24 | 4.13 | 4 | 0.73 | 5.51* | 2 | 1.15 | 1.74 |
| LUNG AND BRONCHUS | 24 | 14.90 | 1.61* | 0 | 1.50 | 0.0 | 8 | 4.85 | 1.65 | 16 | 8.56 | 1.87* |
| OTHER RESP | 2 | 0.23 | 8.54* | 0 | 0.03 | 0.0 | 0 | 0.08 | 0.0 | 2 | 0.13 | 15.96* |

Table 7. Histologic confirmation of multiple primary malignancies

FIRST PRIMARY SITE - LIP

| Subsequent primary site | Both tumors micro-scopically confirmed | | Only 1st tumor micro-scopically confirmed | | Only 2nd tumor micro-scopically confirmed | | Neither tumor micro-scopically confirmed | |
|---|---|---|---|---|---|---|---|---|
| | No. | % | No. | % | No. | % | No. | % |
| LIP | 7 | 100.0 | 0 | 0.0 | 0 | 0.0 | 0 | 0.0 |
| TONGUE | 7 | 77.8 | 0 | 0.0 | 2 | 22.2 | 0 | 0.0 |
| SALIVARY GLAND | 1 | 50.0 | 1 | 50.0 | 0 | 0.0 | 0 | 0.0 |
| MOUTH | 6 | 85.7 | 0 | 0.0 | 0 | 0.0 | 1 | 14.3 |
| LUNG AND BRONCHUS | 13 | 54.2 | 9 | 37.5 | 2 | 8.3 | 0 | 0.0 |
| OTHER RESP | 0 | 0.0 | 2 | 100.0 | 0 | 0.0 | 0 | 0.0 |

Table 8. Subsequent multiple primary malignancies in patients with an index malignant tumor of the tongue

FIRST PRIMARY SITE - TONGUE

| SUBSEQUENT PRIMARY SITES | TOTAL | | | MALES | | | FEMALES | | |
|---|---|---|---|---|---|---|---|---|---|
| | NUMBER OF PERSONS= 1093 PERSON-YRS OF OBSERVATION = 3032.0 | | | NUMBER OF PERSONS= 885 PERSON-YRS OF OBSERVATION = 2280.7 | | | NUMBER OF PERSONS= 208 PERSON-YRS OF OBSERVATION = 751.2 | | |
| | OBS | EXP | OBS/EXP | OBS | EXP | OBS/EXP | OBS | EXP | OBS/EXP |
| LIP | 1 | 0.44 | 2.27 | 1 | 0.43 | 2.33 | 0 | 0.01 | 0.0 |
| TONGUE | 2 | 0.37 | 5.36 | 1 | 0.35 | 2.84 | 1 | 0.02 | 48.53* |
| SALIVARY GLAND | 0 | 0.10 | 0.0 | 0 | 0.08 | 0.0 | 0 | 0.02 | 0.0 |
| MOUTH | 6 | 0.47 | 12.66** | 2 | 0.44 | 4.56 | 4 | 0.04 | 112.10** |
| PHARYNX | 7 | 0.46 | 15.09** | 6 | 0.44 | 13.70** | 1 | 0.03 | 38.76 |
| ESOPHAGUS | 8 | 0.82 | 9.74** | 7 | 0.78 | 9.00** | 1 | 0.04 | 22.70 |
| STOMACH | 4 | 3.23 | 1.24 | 4 | 2.70 | 1.48 | 0 | 0.53 | 0.0 |
| SMALL INTESTINE | 0 | 0.12 | 0.0 | 0 | 0.09 | 0.0 | 0 | 0.03 | 0.0 |
| COLON | 3 | 4.23 | 0.71 | 2 | 3.10 | 0.65 | 1 | 1.13 | 0.88 |
| RECTUM | 3 | 2.48 | 1.21 | 3 | 2.02 | 1.49 | 0 | 0.46 | 0.0 |
| LIVER & BILIARY PASS | 0 | 0.82 | 0.0 | 0 | 0.58 | 0.0 | 0 | 0.24 | 0.0 |
| PANCREAS | 1 | 1.26 | 0.79 | 1 | 1.02 | 0.98 | 0 | 0.24 | 0.0 |
| NOSE AND SINUSES | 0 | 0.07 | 0.0 | 0 | 0.06 | 0.0 | 0 | 0.01 | 0.0 |
| LARYNX | 1 | 0.63 | 1.60 | 1 | 0.61 | 1.63 | 0 | 0.01 | 0.0 |
| LUNG AND BRONCHUS | 6 | 3.54 | 1.69 | 5 | 3.35 | 1.49 | 1 | 0.19 | 5.24 |
| OTHER RESP | 0 | 0.06 | 0.0 | 0 | 0.05 | 0.0 | 0 | 0.01 | 0.0 |
| BREAST | 2 | 1.71 | 1.17 | 0 | 0.07 | 0.0 | 2 | 1.64 | 1.22 |
| CERVIX UTERI | 0 | 0.34 | 0.0 | 0 | 0.0 | 0.0 | 0 | 0.34 | 0.0 |
| CORPUS UTERI | 0 | 0.33 | 0.0 | 0 | 0.0 | 0.0 | 0 | 0.33 | 0.0 |
| UTERUS,UNSPEC | 0 | 0.19 | 0.0 | 0 | 0.0 | 0.0 | 0 | 0.19 | 0.0 |
| OVARY | 0 | 0.31 | 0.0 | 0 | 0.0 | 0.0 | 0 | 0.31 | 0.0 |
| OTHER FEMALE GENITAL | 1 | 0.08 | 12.26 | 0 | 0.0 | 0.0 | 1 | 0.08 | 12.26 |
| PROSTATE | 7 | 4.89 | 1.43 | 7 | 4.89 | 1.43 | 0 | 0.0 | 0.0 |
| TESTIS | 0 | 0.05 | 0.0 | 0 | 0.05 | 0.0 | 0 | 0.0 | 0.0 |
| OTHER MALE GENITAL | 0 | 0.10 | 0.0 | 0 | 0.10 | 0.0 | 0 | 0.0 | 0.0 |
| KIDNEY AND URETER | 2 | 0.70 | 2.87 | 2 | 0.59 | 3.42 | 0 | 0.11 | 0.0 |
| BLADDER | 2 | 2.17 | 0.92 | 1 | 1.93 | 0.52 | 1 | 0.24 | 4.21 |
| MELANOMA OF SKIN | 1 | 0.20 | 4.94 | 1 | 0.15 | 6.64 | 0 | 0.05 | 0.0 |
| EYE | 0 | 0.06 | 0.0 | 0 | 0.05 | 0.0 | 0 | 0.01 | 0.0 |
| NERVOUS SYSTEM | 0 | 0.28 | 0.0 | 0 | 0.22 | 0.0 | 0 | 0.06 | 0.0 |
| THYROID | 1 | 0.12 | 8.00 | 0 | 0.07 | 0.0 | 1 | 0.05 | 19.08 |
| BONE | 0 | 0.09 | 0.0 | 0 | 0.07 | 0.0 | 0 | 0.02 | 0.0 |
| SOFT TISSUE | 0 | 0.21 | 0.0 | 0 | 0.16 | 0.0 | 0 | 0.04 | 0.0 |
| LYMPHOMAS & MYELOMA | 1 | 0.88 | 1.14 | 1 | 0.69 | 1.44 | 0 | 0.19 | 0.0 |
| LEUKEMIAS | 2 | 0.96 | 2.09 | 2 | 0.78 | 2.56 | 0 | 0.18 | 0.0 |
| OTHER SITES | 2 | 1.88 | 1.07 | 2 | 1.42 | 1.41 | 0 | 0.46 | 0.0 |
| TOTAL | 63 | 34.66 | 1.82** | 49 | 27.34 | 1.79** | 14 | 7.33 | 1.91* |

Table 9. Subsequent primary sites with excesses

FIRST PRIMARY SITE - TONGUE

| SUBSEQUENT PRIMARY SITES | TOTAL<br>NUMBER OF PERSONS= 1093<br>PERSON-YRS OF OBSERVATION= 3032.0 | | | YEARS < 1<br>NUMBER OF PERSONS= 1093<br>PERSON-YRS OF OBSERVATION= 862.2 | | | YEARS 1-5<br>NUMBER OF PERSONS= 616<br>PERSON-YRS OF OBSERVATION= 1247.7 | | | YEARS > 5<br>NUMBER OF PERSONS= 189<br>PERSON-YRS OF OBSERVATION= 922.1 | | |
|---|---|---|---|---|---|---|---|---|---|---|---|---|
| | OBS | EXP | OBS/EXP | OBS | EXP | OBS/EXP | OBS | EXP | OBS/EXP | OBS | EXP | OBS/EXP |
| TONGUE | 2 | 0.37 | 5.36 | 0 | 0.11 | 0.0 | 2 | 0.14 | 13.89* | 0 | 0.12 | 0.0 |
| MOUTH | 6 | 0.47 | 12.66** | 1 | 0.13 | 7.63 | 4 | 0.19 | 21.61** | 1 | 0.16 | 6.34 |
| PHARYNX | 7 | 0.46 | 15.09** | 2 | 0.13 | 15.66* | 3 | 0.18 | 16.38** | 2 | 0.15 | 13.07* |
| ESOPHAGUS | 8 | 0.82 | 9.74** | 3 | 0.23 | 13.10** | 4 | 0.32 | 12.47** | 1 | 0.27 | 3.68 |

Table 10. Histologic confirmation of multiple primary malignancies

FIRST PRIMARY SITE - TONGUE

| Subsequent primary site | Both tumors microscopically confirmed | | Only 1st tumor microscopically confirmed | | Only 2nd tumor microscopically confirmed | | Neither tumor microscopically confirmed | |
|---|---|---|---|---|---|---|---|---|
| | No. | % | No. | % | No. | % | No. | % |
| TONGUE | 2 | 100.0 | 0 | 0.0 | 0 | 0.0 | 0 | 0.0 |
| MOUTH | 5 | 83.3 | 0 | 0.0 | 1 | 16.7 | 0 | 0.0 |
| PHARYNX | 7 | 100.0 | 0 | 0.0 | 0 | 0.0 | 0 | 0.0 |
| ESOPHAGUS | 7 | 87.5 | 0 | 0.0 | 1 | 12.5 | 0 | 0.0 |

Table 11. Subsequent multiple primary malignancies in patients with an index malignant tumor of the salivary gland

FIRST PRIMARY SITE - SALIVARY GLAND

| | TOTAL | | | MALES | | | FEMALES | | |
|---|---|---|---|---|---|---|---|---|---|
| | NUMBER OF PERSONS= 436 PERSON-YRS OF OBSERVATION = 2285.7 | | | NUMBER OF PERSONS= 227 PERSON-YRS OF OBSERVATION = 1035.2 | | | NUMBER OF PERSONS= 209 PERSON-YRS OF OBSERVATION = 1250.5 | | |
| SUBSEQUENT PRIMARY SITES | OBS | EXP | OBS/EXP | OBS | EXP | OBS/EXP | OBS | EXP | OBS/EXP |
| LIP | 1 | 0.18 | 5.57 | 1 | 0.17 | 5.88 | 0 | 0.01 | 0.0 |
| TONGUE | 1 | 0.16 | 6.37 | 1 | 0.13 | 7.42 | 0 | 0.02 | 0.0 |
| SALIVARY GLAND | 0 | 0.06 | 0.0 | 0 | 0.03 | 0.0 | 0 | 0.03 | 0.0 |
| MOUTH | 0 | 0.21 | 0.0 | 0 | 0.17 | 0.0 | 0 | 0.04 | 0.0 |
| PHARYNX | 0 | 0.20 | 0.0 | 0 | 0.17 | 0.0 | 0 | 0.03 | 0.0 |
| ESOPHAGUS | 0 | 0.36 | 0.0 | 0 | 0.31 | 0.0 | 0 | 0.05 | 0.0 |
| STOMACH | 1 | 1.59 | 0.63 | 0 | 1.08 | 0.0 | 1 | 0.51 | 1.96 |
| SMALL INTESTINE | 0 | 0.06 | 0.0 | 0 | 0.03 | 0.0 | 0 | 0.03 | 0.0 |
| COLON | 3 | 2.41 | 1.24 | 0 | 1.26 | 0.0 | 3 | 1.16 | 2.60 |
| RECTUM | 2 | 1.31 | 1.52 | 1 | 0.81 | 1.23 | 1 | 0.50 | 2.01 |
| LIVER & BILIARY PASS | 1 | 0.47 | 2.12 | 0 | 0.23 | 0.0 | 1 | 0.24 | 4.18 |
| PANCREAS | 0 | 0.65 | 0.0 | 0 | 0.41 | 0.0 | 0 | 0.25 | 0.0 |
| NOSE AND SINUSES | 0 | 0.04 | 0.0 | 0 | 0.03 | 0.0 | 0 | 0.01 | 0.0 |
| LARYNX | 0 | 0.25 | 0.0 | 0 | 0.23 | 0.0 | 0 | 0.02 | 0.0 |
| LUNG AND BRONCHUS | 2 | 1.46 | 1.37 | 2 | 1.24 | 1.61 | 0 | 0.22 | 0.0 |
| OTHER RESP | 0 | 0.03 | 0.0 | 0 | 0.02 | 0.0 | 0 | 0.01 | 0.0 |
| BREAST | 4 | 2.05 | 1.95 | 1 | 0.03 | 39.67* | 3 | 2.03 | 1.48 |
| CERVIX UTERI | 1 | 0.58 | 1.74 | 0 | 0.0 | 0.0 | 1 | 0.58 | 1.74 |
| CORPUS UTERI | 0 | 0.44 | 0.0 | 0 | 0.0 | 0.0 | 0 | 0.44 | 0.0 |
| UTERUS,UNSPEC | 0 | 0.22 | 0.0 | 0 | 0.0 | 0.0 | 0 | 0.22 | 0.0 |
| OVARY | 0 | 0.41 | 0.0 | 0 | 0.0 | 0.0 | 0 | 0.41 | 0.0 |
| OTHER FEMALE GENITAL | 0 | 0.09 | 0.0 | 0 | 0.0 | 0.0 | 0 | 0.09 | 0.0 |
| PROSTATE | 1 | 2.16 | 0.46 | 1 | 2.16 | 0.46 | 0 | 0.0 | 0.0 |
| TESTIS | 0 | 0.03 | 0.0 | 0 | 0.03 | 0.0 | 0 | 0.0 | 0.0 |
| OTHER MALE GENITAL | 0 | 0.04 | 0.0 | 0 | 0.04 | 0.0 | 0 | 0.0 | 0.0 |
| KIDNEY AND URETER | 0 | 0.35 | 0.0 | 0 | 0.23 | 0.0 | 0 | 0.12 | 0.0 |
| BLADDER | 2 | 1.02 | 1.96 | 0 | 0.79 | 0.0 | 2 | 0.23 | 8.68* |
| MELANOMA OF SKIN | 0 | 0.14 | 0.0 | 0 | 0.07 | 0.0 | 0 | 0.07 | 0.0 |
| EYE | 0 | 0.04 | 0.0 | 0 | 0.02 | 0.0 | 0 | 0.02 | 0.0 |
| NERVOUS SYSTEM | 0 | 0.17 | 0.0 | 0 | 0.08 | 0.0 | 0 | 0.09 | 0.0 |
| THYROID | 0 | 0.10 | 0.0 | 0 | 0.03 | 0.0 | 0 | 0.07 | 0.0 |
| BONE | 0 | 0.05 | 0.0 | 0 | 0.03 | 0.0 | 0 | 0.02 | 0.0 |
| SOFT TISSUE | 0 | 0.12 | 0.0 | 0 | 0.07 | 0.0 | 0 | 0.05 | 0.0 |
| LYMPHOMAS & MYELOMA | 0 | 0.51 | 0.0 | 0 | 0.28 | 0.0 | 0 | 0.23 | 0.0 |
| LEUKEMIAS | 0 | 0.51 | 0.0 | 0 | 0.32 | 0.0 | 0 | 0.20 | 0.0 |
| OTHER SITES | 0 | 1.04 | 0.0 | 0 | 0.57 | 0.0 | 0 | 0.47 | 0.0 |
| TOTAL | 19 | 19.51 | 0.97 | 7 | 11.07 | 0.63 | 12 | 8.44 | 1.42 |

Table 12. Subsequent primary sites with excesses

FIRST PRIMARY SITE - SALIVARY GLAND

| SUBSEQUENT PRIMARY SITES | TOTAL | | | YEARS < 1 | | | YEARS 1-5 | | | YEARS > 5 | | |
|---|---|---|---|---|---|---|---|---|---|---|---|---|
| | NUMBER OF PERSONS= 436<br>PERSON-YRS OF OBSERVATION= 2285.7 | | | NUMBER OF PERSONS= 436<br>PERSON-YRS OF OBSERVATION= 372.8 | | | NUMBER OF PERSONS= 313<br>PERSON-YRS OF OBSERVATION= 891.2 | | | NUMBER OF PERSONS= 167<br>PERSON-YRS OF OBSERVATION= 1021.7 | | |
| | OBS | EXP | OBS/EXP | OBS | EXP | OBS/EXP | OBS | EXP | OBS/EXP | OBS | EXP | OBS/EXP |
| BREAST | 4 | 2.05 | 1.95 | 0 | 0.29 | 0.0 | 3 | 0.74 | 4.05 | 1 | 1.03 | 0.97 |
| BLADDER | 2 | 1.02 | 1.96 | 0 | 0.16 | 0.0 | 1 | 0.35 | 2.82 | 1 | 0.51 | 1.98 |

Table 13. Histologic confirmation of multiple primary malignancies

FIRST PRIMARY SITE - SALIVARY GLAND

| Subsequent primary site | Both tumors microscopically confirmed | | Only 1st tumor microscopically confirmed | | Only 2nd tumor microscopically confirmed | | Neither tumor microscopically confirmed | |
|---|---|---|---|---|---|---|---|---|
| | No. | % | No. | % | No. | % | No. | % |
| BREAST | 2 | 50.0 | 1 | 25.0 | 0 | 0.0 | 1 | 25.0 |
| BLADDER | 0 | 0.0 | 1 | 50.0 | 1 | 50.0 | 0 | 0.0 |

Table 14. Subsequent multiple primary malignancies in patients with an index malignant tumor of the mouth

FIRST PRIMARY SITE - MOUTH

| SUBSEQUENT PRIMARY SITES | TOTAL<br>NUMBER OF PERSONS= 1473<br>PERSON-YRS OF OBSERVATION = 5323.2 | | | MALES<br>NUMBER OF PERSONS= 1165<br>PERSON-YRS OF OBSERVATION = 3939.2 | | | FEMALES<br>NUMBER OF PERSONS= 308<br>PERSON-YRS OF OBSERVATION = 1384.0 | | |
|---|---|---|---|---|---|---|---|---|---|
| | OBS | EXP | OBS/EXP | OBS | EXP | OBS/EXP | OBS | EXP | OBS/EXP |
| LIP | 2 | 0.82 | 2.44 | 2 | 0.81 | 2.48 | 0 | 0.02 | 0.0 |
| TONGUE | 9 | 0.66 | 13.60** | 8 | 0.63 | 12.70** | 1 | 0.03 | 31.45 |
| SALIVARY GLAND | 2 | 0.18 | 11.28* | 1 | 0.15 | 6.88 | 1 | 0.03 | 31.26 |
| MOUTH | 17 | 0.87 | 19.64** | 14 | 0.81 | 17.30** | 3 | 0.06 | 53.13** |
| PHARYNX | 7 | 0.83 | 8.40** | 6 | 0.79 | 7.60** | 1 | 0.04 | 23.02 |
| ESOPHAGUS | 16 | 1.49 | 10.71** | 16 | 1.42 | 11.25** | 0 | 0.07 | 0.0 |
| STOMACH | 8 | 5.82 | 1.37 | 8 | 5.00 | 1.60 | 0 | 0.82 | 0.0 |
| SMALL INTESTINE | 1 | 0.21 | 4.87 | 1 | 0.16 | 6.25 | 0 | 0.05 | 0.0 |
| COLON | 10 | 7.39 | 1.35 | 8 | 5.70 | 1.40 | 2 | 1.69 | 1.19 |
| RECTUM | 4 | 4.41 | 0.91 | 4 | 3.69 | 1.08 | 0 | 0.72 | 0.0 |
| LIVER & BILIARY PASS | 1 | 1.44 | 0.69 | 1 | 1.08 | 0.93 | 0 | 0.36 | 0.0 |
| PANCREAS | 3 | 2.24 | 1.34 | 3 | 1.88 | 1.59 | 0 | 0.36 | 0.0 |
| NOSE AND SINUSES | 1 | 0.13 | 7.61 | 0 | 0.11 | 0.0 | 1 | 0.02 | 59.35* |
| LARYNX | 3 | 1.10 | 2.72 | 2 | 1.08 | 1.85 | 1 | 0.02 | 47.45* |
| LUNG AND BRONCHUS | 16 | 6.20 | 2.58** | 14 | 5.91 | 2.37** | 2 | 0.28 | 7.05 |
| OTHER RESP | 0 | 0.10 | 0.0 | 0 | 0.09 | 0.0 | 0 | 0.01 | 0.0 |
| BREAST | 5 | 2.81 | 1.78 | 0 | 0.12 | 0.0 | 5 | 2.69 | 1.86 |
| CERVIX UTERI | 1 | 0.63 | 1.59 | 0 | 0.0 | 0.0 | 1 | 0.63 | 1.59 |
| CORPUS UTERI | 1 | 0.54 | 1.85 | 0 | 0.0 | 0.0 | 1 | 0.54 | 1.85 |
| UTERUS,UNSPEC | 0 | 0.33 | 0.0 | 0 | 0.0 | 0.0 | 0 | 0.33 | 0.0 |
| OVARY | 0 | 0.51 | 0.0 | 0 | 0.0 | 0.0 | 0 | 0.51 | 0.0 |
| OTHER FEMALE GENITAL | 0 | 0.12 | 0.0 | 0 | 0.0 | 0.0 | 0 | 0.12 | 0.0 |
| PROSTATE | 16 | 9.44 | 1.70 | 16 | 9.44 | 1.70 | 0 | 0.0 | 0.0 |
| TESTIS | 0 | 0.09 | 0.0 | 0 | 0.09 | 0.0 | 0 | 0.0 | 0.0 |
| OTHER MALE GENITAL | 0 | 0.18 | 0.0 | 0 | 0.18 | 0.0 | 0 | 0.0 | 0.0 |
| KIDNEY AND URETER | 2 | 1.21 | 1.66 | 2 | 1.04 | 1.92 | 0 | 0.17 | 0.0 |
| BLADDER | 6 | 3.91 | 1.53 | 6 | 3.57 | 1.68 | 0 | 0.34 | 0.0 |
| MELANOMA OF SKIN | 0 | 0.35 | 0.0 | 0 | 0.27 | 0.0 | 0 | 0.08 | 0.0 |
| EYE | 1 | 0.11 | 9.04 | 0 | 0.09 | 0.0 | 1 | 0.02 | 42.93* |
| NERVOUS SYSTEM | 1 | 0.47 | 2.13 | 0 | 0.36 | 0.0 | 1 | 0.11 | 9.50 |
| THYROID | 1 | 0.21 | 4.73 | 1 | 0.13 | 7.75 | 0 | 0.08 | 0.0 |
| BONE | 0 | 0.16 | 0.0 | 0 | 0.13 | 0.0 | 0 | 0.03 | 0.0 |
| SOFT TISSUE | 0 | 0.36 | 0.0 | 0 | 0.30 | 0.0 | 0 | 0.07 | 0.0 |
| LYMPHOMAS & MYELOMA | 1 | 1.52 | 0.66 | 1 | 1.25 | 0.80 | 0 | 0.28 | 0.0 |
| LEUKEMIAS | 2 | 1.68 | 1.19 | 2 | 1.42 | 1.41 | 0 | 0.26 | 0.0 |
| OTHER SITES | 5 | 3.27 | 1.53 | 4 | 2.61 | 1.54 | 1 | 0.66 | 1.50 |
| TOTAL | 142 | 61.81 | 2.30** | 120 | 50.31 | 2.39** | 22 | 11.49 | 1.91** |

Table 15. Subsequent primary sites with excesses

FIRST PRIMARY SITE - MOUTH

| SUBSEQUENT PRIMARY SITES | TOTAL | | | YEARS < 1 | | | YEARS 1-5 | | | YEARS > 5 | | |
|---|---|---|---|---|---|---|---|---|---|---|---|---|
| | NUMBER OF PERSONS= 1473 PERSON-YRS OF OBSERVATION= 5323.2 | | | NUMBER OF PERSONS= 1473 PERSON-YRS OF OBSERVATION= 1222.2 | | | NUMBER OF PERSONS= 967 PERSON-YRS OF OBSERVATION= 2229.2 | | | NUMBER OF PERSONS= 345 PERSON-YRS OF OBSERVATION= 1871.7 | | |
| | OBS | EXP | OBS/EXP | OBS | EXP | OBS/EXP | OBS | EXP | OBS/EXP | OBS | EXP | OBS/EXP |
| TONGUE | 9 | 0.66 | 13.60** | 2 | 0.15 | 13.06* | 4 | 0.27 | 14.68** | 3 | 0.24 | 12.70** |
| SALIVARY GLAND | 2 | 0.18 | 11.28* | 1 | 0.04 | 25.40 | 1 | 0.07 | 14.31 | 0 | 0.07 | 0.0 |
| MOUTH | 17 | 0.87 | 19.64** | 2 | 0.20 | 10.00* | 6 | 0.35 | 17.16** | 9 | 0.32 | 28.49** |
| PHARYNX | 7 | 0.83 | 8.40** | 0 | 0.19 | 0.0 | 6 | 0.34 | 17.76** | 1 | 0.31 | 3.25 |
| ESOPHAGUS | 16 | 1.49 | 10.71** | 4 | 0.34 | 11.70** | 10 | 0.60 | 16.53** | 2 | 0.55 | 3.66 |
| NOSE AND SINUSES | 1 | 0.13 | 7.61 | 0 | 0.03 | 0.0 | 1 | 0.05 | 19.54 | 0 | 0.05 | 0.0 |
| LARYNX | 3 | 1.10 | 2.72 | 0 | 0.25 | 0.0 | 1 | 0.46 | 2.18 | 2 | 0.40 | 5.04 |
| LUNG AND BRONCHUS | 16 | 6.20 | 2.58** | 1 | 1.32 | 0.76 | 5 | 2.56 | 1.95 | 10 | 2.31 | 4.32** |
| PROSTATE | 16 | 9.44 | 1.70 | 3 | 1.96 | 1.53 | 4 | 3.55 | 1.13 | 9 | 3.92 | 2.29* |
| EYE | 1 | 0.11 | 9.04 | 0 | 0.02 | 0.0 | 1 | 0.04 | 22.28 | 0 | 0.04 | 0.0 |

Table 16. Histologic confirmation of multiple primary malignancies

FIRST PRIMARY SITE - MOUTH

| Subsequent primary site | Both tumors microscopically confirmed | | Only 1st tumor microscopically confirmed | | Only 2nd tumor microscopically confirmed | | Neither tumor microscopically confirmed | |
|---|---|---|---|---|---|---|---|---|
| | No. | % | No. | % | No. | % | No. | % |
| TONGUE | 9 | 100.0 | 0 | 0.0 | 0 | 0.0 | 0 | 0.0 |
| SALIVARY GLAND | 2 | 100.0 | 0 | 0.0 | 0 | 0.0 | 0 | 0.0 |
| MOUTH | 17 | 100.0 | 0 | 0.0 | 0 | 0.0 | 0 | 0.0 |
| PHARYNX | 6 | 85.7 | 1 | 14.3 | 0 | 0.0 | 0 | 0.0 |
| ESOPHAGUS | 15 | 93.8 | 1 | 6.3 | 0 | 0.0 | 0 | 0.0 |
| NOSE AND SINUSES | 1 | 100.0 | 0 | 0.0 | 0 | 0.0 | 0 | 0.0 |
| LARYNX | 2 | 66.7 | 0 | 0.0 | 1 | 33.3 | 0 | 0.0 |
| LUNG AND BRONCHUS | 12 | 75.0 | 3 | 18.8 | 0 | 0.0 | 1 | 6.3 |
| PROSTATE | 14 | 87.5 | 2 | 12.5 | 0 | 0.0 | 0 | 0.0 |
| EYE | 1 | 100.0 | 0 | 0.0 | 0 | 0.0 | 0 | 0.0 |

Table 17. Subsequent multiple primary malignancies in patients with an index malignant tumor of the pharynx

FIRST PRIMARY SITE - PHARYNX

| SUBSEQUENT PRIMARY SITES | TOTAL<br>NUMBER OF PERSONS= 1386<br>PERSON-YRS OF OBSERVATION = 3149.9<br>OBS | EXP | OBS/EXP | MALES<br>NUMBER OF PERSONS= 1117<br>PERSON-YRS OF OBSERVATION = 2323.0<br>OBS | EXP | OBS/EXP | FEMALES<br>NUMBER OF PERSONS= 269<br>PERSON-YRS OF OBSERVATION = 826.9<br>OBS | EXP | OBS/EXP |
|---|---|---|---|---|---|---|---|---|---|
| LIP | 2 | 0.40 | 5.05 | 2 | 0.39 | 5.15 | 0 | 0.01 | 0.0 |
| TONGUE | 9 | 0.34 | 26.17** | 9 | 0.33 | 27.44** | 0 | 0.02 | 0.0 |
| SALIVARY GLAND | 0 | 0.09 | 0.0 | 0 | 0.07 | 0.0 | 0 | 0.02 | 0.0 |
| MOUTH | 8 | 0.43 | 18.47** | 7 | 0.41 | 17.22** | 1 | 0.03 | 37.78 |
| PHARYNX | 6 | 0.45 | 13.48** | 6 | 0.42 | 14.27** | 0 | 0.02 | 0.0 |
| ESOPHAGUS | 7 | 0.78 | 8.98** | 7 | 0.74 | 9.43** | 0 | 0.04 | 0.0 |
| STOMACH | 8 | 2.85 | 2.81* | 6 | 2.45 | 2.45 | 2 | 0.40 | 5.03 |
| SMALL INTESTINE | 0 | 0.11 | 0.0 | 0 | 0.09 | 0.0 | 0 | 0.02 | 0.0 |
| COLON | 5 | 3.69 | 1.35 | 4 | 2.85 | 1.41 | 1 | 0.85 | 1.18 |
| RECTUM | 3 | 2.23 | 1.35 | 3 | 1.86 | 1.61 | 0 | 0.37 | 0.0 |
| LIVER & BILIARY PASS | 2 | 0.72 | 2.78 | 1 | 0.53 | 1.87 | 1 | 0.18 | 5.44 |
| PANCREAS | 1 | 1.12 | 0.89 | 1 | 0.94 | 1.07 | 0 | 0.18 | 0.0 |
| NOSE AND SINUSES | 0 | 0.07 | 0.0 | 0 | 0.06 | 0.0 | 0 | 0.01 | 0.0 |
| LARYNX | 1 | 0.61 | 1.65 | 1 | 0.60 | 1.68 | 0 | 0.01 | 0.0 |
| LUNG AND BRONCHUS | 8 | 3.52 | 2.27 | 8 | 3.37 | 2.38* | 0 | 0.15 | 0.0 |
| OTHER RESP | 0 | 0.06 | 0.0 | 0 | 0.05 | 0.0 | 0 | 0.00 | 0.0 |
| BREAST | 2 | 1.50 | 1.33 | 0 | 0.07 | 0.0 | 2 | 1.44 | 1.39 |
| CERVIX UTERI | 0 | 0.38 | 0.0 | 0 | 0.0 | 0.0 | 0 | 0.38 | 0.0 |
| CORPUS UTERI | 1 | 0.31 | 3.23 | 0 | 0.0 | 0.0 | 1 | 0.31 | 3.23 |
| UTERUS,UNSPEC | 0 | 0.18 | 0.0 | 0 | 0.0 | 0.0 | 0 | 0.18 | 0.0 |
| OVARY | 0 | 0.29 | 0.0 | 0 | 0.0 | 0.0 | 0 | 0.29 | 0.0 |
| OTHER FEMALE GENITAL | 0 | 0.06 | 0.0 | 0 | 0.0 | 0.0 | 0 | 0.06 | 0.0 |
| PROSTATE | 8 | 4.22 | 1.90 | 8 | 4.22 | 1.90 | 0 | 0.0 | 0.0 |
| TESTIS | 1 | 0.05 | 18.69 | 1 | 0.05 | 18.69 | 0 | 0.0 | 0.0 |
| OTHER MALE GENITAL | 0 | 0.09 | 0.0 | 0 | 0.09 | 0.0 | 0 | 0.0 | 0.0 |
| KIDNEY AND URETER | 1 | 0.65 | 1.53 | 1 | 0.56 | 1.77 | 0 | 0.09 | 0.0 |
| BLADDER | 0 | 1.95 | 0.0 | 0 | 1.78 | 0.0 | 0 | 0.17 | 0.0 |
| MELANOMA OF SKIN | 1 | 0.19 | 5.25 | 0 | 0.14 | 0.0 | 1 | 0.05 | 20.52 |
| EYE | 0 | 0.06 | 0.0 | 0 | 0.05 | 0.0 | 0 | 0.01 | 0.0 |
| NERVOUS SYSTEM | 0 | 0.29 | 0.0 | 0 | 0.23 | 0.0 | 0 | 0.06 | 0.0 |
| THYROID | 0 | 0.11 | 0.0 | 0 | 0.07 | 0.0 | 0 | 0.05 | 0.0 |
| BONE | 0 | 0.08 | 0.0 | 0 | 0.06 | 0.0 | 0 | 0.02 | 0.0 |
| SOFT TISSUE | 1 | 0.20 | 5.07 | 1 | 0.16 | 6.26 | 0 | 0.04 | 0.0 |
| LYMPHOMAS & MYELOMA | 2 | 0.83 | 2.42 | 2 | 0.67 | 2.99 | 0 | 0.16 | 0.0 |
| LEUKEMIAS | 2 | 0.88 | 2.26 | 2 | 0.74 | 2.69 | 0 | 0.14 | 0.0 |
| OTHER SITES | 3 | 1.66 | 1.81 | 2 | 1.33 | 1.51 | 1 | 0.34 | 2.98 |
| TOTAL | 82 | 31.44 | 2.61** | 72 | 25.37 | 2.84** | 10 | 6.08 | 1.65 |

Table 18. Subsequent primary sites with excesses

FIRST PRIMARY SITE - PHARYNX

| SUBSEQUENT PRIMARY SITES | TOTAL | | | YEARS < 1 | | | YEARS 1-5 | | | YEARS > 5 | | |
|---|---|---|---|---|---|---|---|---|---|---|---|---|
| | NUMBER OF PERSONS= 1386 PERSON-YRS OF OBSERVATION= 3149.9 | | | NUMBER OF PERSONS= 1386 PERSON-YRS OF OBSERVATION= 1020.5 | | | NUMBER OF PERSONS= 698 PERSON-YRS OF OBSERVATION= 1331.3 | | | NUMBER OF PERSONS= 171 PERSON-YRS OF OBSERVATION= 798.1 | | |
| | OBS | EXP | OBS/EXP | OBS | EXP | OBS/EXP | OBS | EXP | OBS/EXP | OBS | EXP | OBS/EXP |
| TONGUE | 9 | 0.34 | 26.17** | 7 | 0.11 | 62.22** | 1 | 0.14 | 6.92 | 1 | 0.09 | 11.52 |
| MOUTH | 8 | 0.43 | 18.47** | 3 | 0.14 | 21.14** | 4 | 0.18 | 22.39** | 1 | 0.11 | 8.89 |
| PHARYNX | 6 | 0.45 | 13.48** | 1 | 0.15 | 6.72 | 3 | 0.19 | 16.20** | 2 | 0.11 | 18.00* |
| ESOPHAGUS | 7 | 0.78 | 8.98** | 2 | 0.25 | 7.91 | 4 | 0.32 | 12.38** | 1 | 0.20 | 4.91 |
| STOMACH | 8 | 2.85 | 2.81* | 4 | 0.92 | 4.34* | 3 | 1.18 | 2.55 | 1 | 0.75 | 1.33 |
| LUNG AND BRONCHUS | 8 | 3.52 | 2.27 | 2 | 1.11 | 1.80 | 3 | 1.50 | 2.00 | 3 | 0.91 | 3.31 |
| TESTIS | 1 | 0.05 | 18.69 | 0 | 0.02 | 0.0 | 1 | 0.02 | 44.38* | 0 | 0.01 | 0.0 |
| OTHER SITES | 3 | 1.66 | 1.81 | 3 | 0.50 | 6.00* | 0 | 0.70 | 0.0 | 0 | 0.46 | 0.0 |

Table 19. Histologic confirmation of multiple primary malignancies

FIRST PRIMARY SITE - PHARYNX

| Subsequent primary site | Both tumors microscopically confirmed | | Only 1st tumor microscopically confirmed | | Only 2nd tumor microscopically confirmed | | Neither tumor microscopically confirmed | |
|---|---|---|---|---|---|---|---|---|
| | No. | % | No. | % | No. | % | No. | % |
| TONGUE | 9 | 100.0 | 0 | 0.0 | 0 | 0.0 | 0 | 0.0 |
| MOUTH | 7 | 87.5 | 0 | 0.0 | 1 | 12.5 | 0 | 0.0 |
| PHARYNX | 5 | 83.3 | 0 | 0.0 | 0 | 0.0 | 1 | 16.7 |
| ESOPHAGUS | 6 | 85.7 | 0 | 0.0 | 0 | 0.0 | 1 | 14.3 |
| STOMACH | 6 | 75.0 | 2 | 25.0 | 0 | 0.0 | 0 | 0.0 |
| LUNG AND BRONCHUS | 6 | 75.0 | 2 | 25.0 | 0 | 0.0 | 0 | 0.0 |
| TESTIS | 1 | 100.0 | 0 | 0.0 | 0 | 0.0 | 0 | 0.0 |
| OTHER SITES | 3 | 100.0 | 0 | 0.0 | 0 | 0.0 | 0 | 0.0 |

Table 20. Summary of site-group pairs with an excess of observed-over-expected subsequent primary malignancies: index tumors of the buccal cavity and pharynx

I. Possibly artifact

- Pharynx ◄──────► Testis
- Salivary gland ──────► Bladder
- Mouth ──────► Prostate
- Mouth ──────► Eye
- Pharynx ──────► Other/unspecified sites

II. Possibly real

A. In organs within the same system

1. Same or paired organs

- Lip ◄──────► Lip
- Tongue ◄──────► Tongue
- Mouth ◄──────► Mouth
- Pharynx ◄──────► Pharynx

2. Others

- Tongue ◄──────► Mouth
- Tongue ◄──────► Pharynx
- Mouth ◄──────► Pharynx
- Mouth ──────► Salivary gland
- Lip ──────► Tongue
- Lip ──────► Salivary gland
- Lip ──────► Mouth

B. In organs related structurally or functionally

- Mouth ◄──────► Esophagus
- Lip ──────► Lung/bronchus
- Lip ──────► Other respiratory
- Tongue ──────► Esophagus
- Mouth ──────► Nose and sinuses
- Mouth ──────► Larynx
- Mouth ──────► Lung/bronchus
- Pharynx ──────► Esophagus
- Pharynx ──────► Stomach
- Pharynx ──────► Lung/bronchus

C. In organs apparently unrelated structurally or functionally

- Salivary gland ──────► Breast

Table 21. Common metastatic sites for primary malignant tumors of the buccal cavity and pharynx (HOLLAND and FREI, 1973; WILLIS, 1973; RUBIN, 1974)

| Anatomic location of the primary malignant tumor | Common metastatic sites |
|---|---|
| Lip and oral cavity | Submental, facial, and cervical lymph nodes; mandible; liver; lung; base of skull and cranial nerves |
| Salivary glands | Lung; middle ear; base of brain |

# Chapter 7

# Index Tumors of the Digestive System

Population Studied. 19,158 males and 15,893 females with cancer of the digestive system were followed for the subsequent development of independent primary malignant neoplasms; 1,125 such subsequent neoplasms were discovered. The cohort of individuals with cancer of the digestive system contributed 83,479 person-years of observation.

Results. Detailed tabulations by site are presented in Tables 22-45. The reader is referred to Chapter 5 for a general explanation of the items in these tables.

Summary of Findings. Site-group pairs with a statistically significant excess of observed-over-expected subsequent primary cancers are categorized in Table 46 on the basis of possible relationships between the anatomic sites containing these cancers. In addition, possible artifactual relationships, based on a small number of cases and with no confirmation from other published reports, are emphasized. Table 47 outlines site-group pairs with a statistically significant deficiency of observed-over-expected subsequent primary cancers.

Discussion. Table 48 presents the common metastatic sites for cancers arising within the digestive system. These data used in conjunction with the site-specific tabulations of the percentage of multiple primary malignancies with histologic confirmation, are useful in distinguishing real from artifactual associations.

The relationships noted in the first category are thought to be spurious. As noted in Chapter 4, prostatic cancer frequently appears in excess in patients with cancers of other sites. Cancer patients who die are more likely to come to autopsy than the general population of deaths. The autopsy examination often discovers the presence of a clinically asymptomatic malignancy. This phenomenon is thought to account for the excess of subsequent prostatic cancer among patients with index malignancies of the digestive system.

The excess of ovarian cancer in women with an index cancer of the small intestine is based on only three cases, and in one instance the intestinal cancer did not have histologic confirmation. The remaining associations noted in group I are based on two or fewer cases and do not have general confirmation in the published literature. Despite the small numbers and lack of confirmation, the association between pancreatic cancer and malignancies of either the pharynx or respiratory system may be related to a common carcinogen. One study has suggested that cigarette smoking, besides increasing the risk of oral cavity and respiratory cancer, also results in an increase in pancreatic cancer (HAMMOND, 1975). Also of interest is the excess of leukemia in patients with an index cancer of the small intestine; for the two patients illustrating this phenomenon, the leukemia was diagnosed 5 or more years after the intestinal malignancy. The patient with cancer of both the pancreas and thyroid may represent multiple endocrine adenomatosis.

Excesses of observed-over-expected subsequent primary cancers occurring in paired organs, in organs within the same system, or in structurally or functionally related organs (categories IIA, IIB, and IIC) may be explained on the basis of related tissue exposed to the same oncogenic factor(s). Multiple primary cancers involving various organs within the digestive system are well-documented in the literature (POLK et al., 1965; MOERTEL, 1966; SCHOTTENFELD et al., 1969; BERG et al., 1970; TRAVIESO et al., 1972; NEWELL et al., 1975). Although for the Connecticut experience the number of observed cases of multiple primary cancers involving the digestive system is sometimes small (e.g., one case of multiple primaries of the esophagus), this occurrence is confirmed by many other investigations and is felt to be a real phenomenon.

The association among cancers of the buccal cavity, pharynx, respiratory system, and upper digestive system has already been discussed in Chapter 6. Some authors (SCHOTTENFELD et al., 1974) have suggested that smoking and alcohol consumption may be important factors in the etiology of this constellation of tumors.

The excess of mouth cancer in colon cancer patients remains unexplained. The anatomic sites involved in this association are at opposite ends of the alimentary canal, and thus could be exposed to a common oncogenic factor. This relationship, however, has yet to be confirmed by more definitive studies. In all seven patients with mouth cancer following colon cancer, both malignancies were microscopically verified.

In organs apparently unrelated functionally or anatomically the following site-group pairs revealed a two-way association:

uterine corpus and colon
ovary and colon

These findings are in agreement with the experience of the Memorial Hospital for Cancer and Allied Diseases (SCHOTTENFELD et al., 1969) and Charity Hospital (NEWELL et al., 1975). They reported an association between carcinoma of the colon and cancer of the female genital organs. It should be pointed out that these results are from single institutions, and the possibility of selection bias in terms of the patient population served by these hospitals must be considered. The present findings from a statewide population-based registry add support to the possible etiologic significance of the findings of these other reports.

A number of investigations of cancer occurrence among members of the same family have revealed a high intrafamilial incidence of gastrointestinal and endometrial cancer (HAUSER and WELLER, 1936; SAVAGE, 1956; LYNCH et al., 1967). Other studies have shown that women with endometrial cancer and colon cancer have a higher frequency of infertility, than might be expected from the general population (SPEERT, 1949; SOMMERS et al., 1949; DOCKERTY et al., 1955; CORSCADEN, 1962; ACHESON et al., submitted for publication). A report of the role of marital status in cancer mortality revealed that nuns have an increased death rate from malignancies affecting the large intestine, breast, uterine corpus, and ovary (FRAUMENI et al., 1969). The relationship between rectal cancer and ovarian malignancies may be on a similar basis. This association is also reported in published tabulations from Charity Hospital in New Orleans (NEWELL et al., 1975).

The excess risk of soft-tissue malignancies in patients with stomach cancer is not supported by the findings of other studies. In all three patients exhibiting such tumors, both neoplasms had histologic confirmation. Whether this association has a biologic basis remains to be determined.

The excess risk of urinary tract cancer in patients with colon cancer is supported by the analysis of the experience of the Memorial Hospital for Cancer and Allied Diseases (SCHOTTENFELD et al., 1969). The excess was not statistically significant. The close anatomic proximity of the colon and urinary tract necessitates careful study to distinguish primary and metastatic lesions. For the Connecticut patients with malignancies of both the large intestine and urinary tract, the two neoplasms were microscopically verified in slightly over 85% of the cases.

With regard to deficiencies of observed-over-expected second primary cancers, those involving the same organ are artifactual. For example, as a treatment for cancer of the stomach or rectum, the entire organ is often removed surgically and the patient is no longer at risk for developing a subsequent cancer of this same organ. Multicentric tumors originating in a single organ and diagnosed at the same time are noted in Chapter 3.

The other deficiencies shown in Table 47 are as yet not supported by other studies and remain of unknown biologic significance.

Table 22. Subsequent multiple primary malignancies in patients with an index malignant tumor of the esophagus

FIRST PRIMARY SITE - ESOPHAGUS

| SUBSEQUENT PRIMARY SITES | TOTAL | | | MALES | | | FEMALES | | |
|---|---|---|---|---|---|---|---|---|---|
| | NUMBER OF PERSONS= 1828<br>PERSON-YRS OF OBSERVATION = 1209.2 | | | NUMBER OF PERSONS= 1529<br>PERSON-YRS OF OBSERVATION = 913.1 | | | NUMBER OF PERSONS= 299<br>PERSON-YRS OF OBSERVATION = 296.1 | | |
| | OBS | EXP | OBS/EXP | OBS | EXP | OBS/EXP | OBS | EXP | OBS/EXP |
| LIP | 1 | 0.18 | 5.69 | 1 | 0.17 | 5.83 | 0 | 0.00 | 0.0 |
| TONGUE | 0 | 0.15 | 0.0 | 0 | 0.14 | 0.0 | 0 | 0.01 | 0.0 |
| SALIVARY GLAND | 0 | 0.04 | 0.0 | 0 | 0.03 | 0.0 | 0 | 0.01 | 0.0 |
| MOUTH | 2 | 0.19 | 10.42* | 2 | 0.18 | 11.32* | 0 | 0.02 | 0.0 |
| PHARYNX | 0 | 0.19 | 0.0 | 0 | 0.18 | 0.0 | 0 | 0.01 | 0.0 |
| ESOPHAGUS | 1 | 0.35 | 2.84 | 0 | 0.33 | 0.0 | 1 | 0.02 | 45.84* |
| STOMACH | 1 | 1.31 | 0.76 | 1 | 1.07 | 0.94 | 0 | 0.24 | 0.0 |
| SMALL INTESTINE | 0 | 0.05 | 0.0 | 0 | 0.04 | 0.0 | 0 | 0.01 | 0.0 |
| COLON | 2 | 1.69 | 1.18 | 2 | 1.22 | 1.64 | 0 | 0.47 | 0.0 |
| RECTUM | 0 | 1.00 | 0.0 | 0 | 0.81 | 0.0 | 0 | 0.19 | 0.0 |
| LIVER & BILIARY PASS | 1 | 0.34 | 2.91 | 1 | 0.23 | 4.27 | 0 | 0.11 | 0.0 |
| PANCREAS | 0 | 0.50 | 0.0 | 0 | 0.40 | 0.0 | 0 | 0.10 | 0.0 |
| NOSE AND SINUSES | 0 | 0.03 | 0.0 | 0 | 0.02 | 0.0 | 0 | 0.00 | 0.0 |
| LARYNX | 1 | 0.26 | 3.81 | 0 | 0.26 | 0.0 | 1 | 0.01 | 199.71** |
| LUNG AND BRONCHUS | 1 | 1.54 | 0.65 | 1 | 1.46 | 0.68 | 0 | 0.07 | 0.0 |
| OTHER RESP | 0 | 0.02 | 0.0 | 0 | 0.02 | 0.0 | 0 | 0.00 | 0.0 |
| BREAST | 0 | 0.71 | 0.0 | 0 | 0.03 | 0.0 | 0 | 0.68 | 0.0 |
| CERVIX UTERI | 0 | 0.13 | 0.0 | 0 | 0.0 | 0.0 | 0 | 0.13 | 0.0 |
| CORPUS UTERI | 0 | 0.13 | 0.0 | 0 | 0.0 | 0.0 | 0 | 0.13 | 0.0 |
| UTERUS,UNSPEC | 0 | 0.09 | 0.0 | 0 | 0.0 | 0.0 | 0 | 0.09 | 0.0 |
| OVARY | 1 | 0.12 | 8.07 | 0 | 0.0 | 0.0 | 1 | 0.12 | 8.07 |
| OTHER FEMALE GENITAL | 0 | 0.03 | 0.0 | 0 | 0.0 | 0.0 | 0 | 0.03 | 0.0 |
| PROSTATE | 4 | 1.81 | 2.21 | 4 | 1.81 | 2.21 | 0 | 0.0 | 0.0 |
| TESTIS | 0 | 0.02 | 0.0 | 0 | 0.02 | 0.0 | 0 | 0.0 | 0.0 |
| OTHER MALE GENITAL | 0 | 0.04 | 0.0 | 0 | 0.04 | 0.0 | 0 | 0.0 | 0.0 |
| KIDNEY AND URETER | 1 | 0.29 | 3.50 | 1 | 0.24 | 4.11 | 0 | 0.04 | 0.0 |
| BLADDER | 0 | 0.87 | 0.0 | 0 | 0.78 | 0.0 | 0 | 0.09 | 0.0 |
| MELANOMA OF SKIN | 0 | 0.08 | 0.0 | 0 | 0.06 | 0.0 | 0 | 0.02 | 0.0 |
| EYE | 0 | 0.03 | 0.0 | 0 | 0.02 | 0.0 | 0 | 0.01 | 0.0 |
| NERVOUS SYSTEM | 0 | 0.12 | 0.0 | 0 | 0.10 | 0.0 | 0 | 0.02 | 0.0 |
| THYROID | 1 | 0.05 | 19.22 | 1 | 0.03 | 33.54 | 0 | 0.02 | 0.0 |
| BONE | 0 | 0.04 | 0.0 | 0 | 0.03 | 0.0 | 0 | 0.01 | 0.0 |
| SOFT TISSUE | 0 | 0.08 | 0.0 | 0 | 0.07 | 0.0 | 0 | 0.02 | 0.0 |
| LYMPHOMAS & MYELOMA | 0 | 0.35 | 0.0 | 0 | 0.28 | 0.0 | 0 | 0.07 | 0.0 |
| LEUKEMIAS | 0 | 0.39 | 0.0 | 0 | 0.32 | 0.0 | 0 | 0.07 | 0.0 |
| OTHER SITES | 1 | 0.75 | 1.33 | 1 | 0.57 | 1.76 | 0 | 0.18 | 0.0 |
| TOTAL | 18 | 13.98 | 1.29 | 15 | 10.96 | 1.37 | 3 | 3.02 | 0.99 |

Table 23. Subsequent primary sites with excesses

FIRST PRIMARY SITE - ESOPHAGUS

| SUBSEQUENT PRIMARY SITES | TOTAL | | | YEARS < 1 | | | YEARS 1-5 | | | YEARS > 5 | | |
|---|---|---|---|---|---|---|---|---|---|---|---|---|
| | NUMBER OF PERSONS= 1828 PERSON-YRS OF OBSERVATION= 1209.2 | | | NUMBER OF PERSONS= 1828 PERSON-YRS OF OBSERVATION= 817.2 | | | NUMBER OF PERSONS= 287 PERSON-YRS OF OBSERVATION= 303.3 | | | NUMBER OF PERSONS= 27 PERSON-YRS OF OBSERVATION= 88.7 | | |
| | OBS | EXP | OBS/EXP | OBS | EXP | OBS/EXP | OBS | EXP | OBS/EXP | OBS | EXP | OBS/EXP |
| LIP | 1 | 0.18 | 5.69 | 0 | 0.13 | 0.0 | 0 | 0.04 | 0.0 | 1 | 0.01 | 130.72* |
| MOUTH | 2 | 0.19 | 10.42* | 2 | 0.14 | 14.65* | 0 | 0.04 | 0.0 | 0 | 0.01 | 0.0 |
| ESOPHAGUS | 1 | 0.35 | 2.84 | 0 | 0.25 | 0.0 | 1 | 0.08 | 12.33 | 0 | 0.02 | 0.0 |
| LARYNX | 1 | 0.26 | 3.81 | 1 | 0.19 | 5.30 | 0 | 0.06 | 0.0 | 0 | 0.01 | 0.0 |

Table 24. Histologic confirmation of multiple primary malignancies

FIRST PRIMARY SITE - ESOPHAGUS

| Subsequent primary site | Both tumors microscopically confirmed | | Only 1st tumor microscopically confirmed | | Only 2nd tumor microscopically confirmed | | Neither tumor microscopically confirmed | |
|---|---|---|---|---|---|---|---|---|
| | No. | % | No. | % | No. | % | No. | % |
| LIP | 1 | 100.0 | 0 | 0.0 | 0 | 0.0 | 0 | 0.0 |
| MOUTH | 2 | 100.0 | 0 | 0.0 | 0 | 0.0 | 0 | 0.0 |
| ESOPHAGUS | 1 | 100.0 | 0 | 0.0 | 0 | 0.0 | 0 | 0.0 |
| LARYNX | 1 | 100.0 | 0 | 0.0 | 0 | 0.0 | 0 | 0.0 |

Table 25. Subsequent multiple primary malignancies in patients with an index malignant tumor of the stomach

FIRST PRIMARY SITE - STOMACH

| | TOTAL | | | MALES | | | FEMALES | | |
|---|---|---|---|---|---|---|---|---|---|
| | NUMBER OF PERSONS= 7496<br>PERSON-YRS OF OBSERVATION = 10343.9 | | | NUMBER OF PERSONS= 4765<br>PERSON-YRS OF OBSERVATION = 6584.2 | | | NUMBER OF PERSONS= 2731<br>PERSON-YRS OF OBSERVATION = 3759.7 | | |
| SUBSEQUENT PRIMARY SITES | OBS | EXP | OBS/EXP | OBS | EXP | OBS/EXP | OBS | EXP | OBS/EXP |
| LIP | 1 | 1.29 | 0.78 | 1 | 1.23 | 0.81 | 0 | 0.05 | 0.0 |
| TONGUE | 1 | 1.10 | 0.91 | 1 | 1.00 | 1.00 | 0 | 0.10 | 0.0 |
| SALIVARY GLAND | 0 | 0.34 | 0.0 | 0 | 0.23 | 0.0 | 0 | 0.11 | 0.0 |
| MOUTH | 1 | 1.44 | 0.70 | 1 | 1.25 | 0.80 | 0 | 0.19 | 0.0 |
| PHARYNX | 1 | 1.40 | 0.71 | 1 | 1.27 | 0.79 | 0 | 0.13 | 0.0 |
| ESOPHAGUS | 2 | 2.55 | 0.78 | 1 | 2.31 | 0.43 | 1 | 0.24 | 4.19 |
| STOMACH | 1 | 10.62 | 0.09** | 1 | 7.73 | 0.13** | 0 | 2.88 | 0.0 |
| SMALL INTESTINE | 0 | 0.42 | 0.0 | 0 | 0.27 | 0.0 | 0 | 0.15 | 0.0 |
| COLON | 16 | 14.84 | 1.08 | 9 | 8.97 | 1.00 | 7 | 5.87 | 1.19 |
| RECTUM | 6 | 8.29 | 0.72 | 5 | 5.88 | 0.85 | 1 | 2.41 | 0.41 |
| LIVER & BILIARY PASS | 4 | 2.98 | 1.34 | 4 | 1.67 | 2.40 | 0 | 1.31 | 0.0 |
| PANCREAS | 2 | 4.26 | 0.47 | 1 | 2.94 | 0.34 | 1 | 1.32 | 0.76 |
| NOSE AND SINUSES | 1 | 0.24 | 4.21 | 1 | 0.17 | 5.76 | 0 | 0.06 | 0.0 |
| LARYNX | 1 | 1.87 | 0.53 | 1 | 1.81 | 0.55 | 0 | 0.06 | 0.0 |
| LUNG AND BRONCHUS | 8 | 11.36 | 0.70 | 7 | 10.39 | 0.67 | 1 | 0.97 | 1.03 |
| OTHER RESP | 0 | 0.19 | 0.0 | 0 | 0.16 | 0.0 | 0 | 0.03 | 0.0 |
| BREAST | 9 | 8.58 | 1.05 | 1 | 0.19 | 5.23 | 8 | 8.39 | 0.95 |
| CERVIX UTERI | 1 | 1.67 | 0.60 | 0 | 0.0 | 0.0 | 1 | 1.67 | 0.60 |
| CORPUS UTERI | 2 | 1.68 | 1.19 | 0 | 0.0 | 0.0 | 2 | 1.68 | 1.19 |
| UTERUS,UNSPEC | 0 | 1.04 | 0.0 | 0 | 0.0 | 0.0 | 0 | 1.04 | 0.0 |
| OVARY | 3 | 1.55 | 1.94 | 0 | 0.0 | 0.0 | 3 | 1.55 | 1.94 |
| OTHER FEMALE GENITAL | 1 | 0.44 | 2.30 | 0 | 0.0 | 0.0 | 1 | 0.44 | 2.30 |
| PROSTATE | 20 | 13.64 | 1.47 | 20 | 13.64 | 1.47 | 0 | 0.0 | 0.0 |
| TESTIS | 0 | 0.15 | 0.0 | 0 | 0.15 | 0.0 | 0 | 0.0 | 0.0 |
| OTHER MALE GENITAL | 0 | 0.28 | 0.0 | 0 | 0.28 | 0.0 | 0 | 0.0 | 0.0 |
| KIDNEY AND URETER | 4 | 2.31 | 1.73 | 3 | 1.74 | 1.73 | 1 | 0.57 | 1.76 |
| BLADDER | 10 | 6.88 | 1.45 | 8 | 5.65 | 1.42 | 2 | 1.23 | 1.62 |
| MELANOMA OF SKIN | 0 | 0.67 | 0.0 | 0 | 0.42 | 0.0 | 0 | 0.25 | 0.0 |
| EYE | 1 | 0.22 | 4.62 | 1 | 0.14 | 7.17 | 0 | 0.08 | 0.0 |
| NERVOUS SYSTEM | 0 | 0.95 | 0.0 | 0 | 0.66 | 0.0 | 0 | 0.29 | 0.0 |
| THYROID | 1 | 0.49 | 2.03 | 0 | 0.22 | 0.0 | 1 | 0.28 | 3.62 |
| BONE | 0 | 0.30 | 0.0 | 0 | 0.19 | 0.0 | 0 | 0.10 | 0.0 |
| SOFT TISSUE | 3 | 0.70 | 4.26 | 3 | 0.49 | 6.12* | 0 | 0.21 | 0.0 |
| LYMPHOMAS & MYELOMA | 1 | 3.00 | 0.33 | 0 | 2.06 | 0.0 | 1 | 0.94 | 1.07 |
| LEUKEMIAS | 3 | 3.25 | 0.92 | 3 | 2.32 | 1.29 | 0 | 0.93 | 0.0 |
| OTHER SITES | 3 | 6.59 | 0.46 | 3 | 4.21 | 0.71 | 0 | 2.38 | 0.0 |
| TOTAL | 107 | 117.57 | 0.91 | 76 | 79.65 | 0.95 | 31 | 37.92 | 0.82 |

Table 26. Subsequent primary sites with excesses

FIRST PRIMARY SITE - STOMACH

| | TOTAL | | | YEARS < 1 | | | YEARS 1-5 | | | YEARS > 5 | | |
|---|---|---|---|---|---|---|---|---|---|---|---|---|
| | NUMBER OF PERSONS= 7496 PERSON-YRS OF OBSERVATION= 10343.9 | | | NUMBER OF PERSONS= 7496 PERSON-YRS OF OBSERVATION= 3808.5 | | | NUMBER OF PERSONS= 2113 PERSON-YRS OF OBSERVATION= 3738.0 | | | NUMBER OF PERSONS= 497 PERSON-YRS OF OBSERVATION= 2797.4 | | |
| SUBSEQUENT PRIMARY SITES | OBS | EXP | OBS/EXP | OBS | EXP | OBS/EXP | OBS | EXP | OBS/EXP | OBS | EXP | OBS/EXP |
| SOFT TISSUE | 3 | 0.70 | 4.26 | 1 | 0.23 | 4.38 | 1 | 0.24 | 4.19 | 1 | 0.24 | 4.22 |

Table 27. Subsequent primary sites with deficiencies

FIRST PRIMARY SITE - STOMACH

| | TOTAL | | | YEARS < 1 | | | YEARS 1-5 | | | YEARS > 5 | | |
|---|---|---|---|---|---|---|---|---|---|---|---|---|
| | NUMBER OF PERSONS= 7496 PERSON-YRS OF OBSERVATION= 10343.9 | | | NUMBER OF PERSONS= 7496 PERSON-YRS OF OBSERVATION= 3808.5 | | | NUMBER OF PERSONS= 2113 PERSON-YRS OF OBSERVATION= 3738.0 | | | NUMBER OF PERSONS= 497 PERSON-YRS OF OBSERVATION= 2797.4 | | |
| SUBSEQUENT PRIMARY SITES | OBS | EXP | OBS/EXP | OBS | EXP | OBS/EXP | OBS | EXP | OBS/EXP | OBS | EXP | OBS/EXP |
| STOMACH | 1 | 10.62 | 0.09** | 0 | 3.78 | 0.0 | 1 | 3.60 | 0.28 | 0 | 3.24 | 0.0 |

Table 28. Histologic confirmation of multiple primary malignancies

FIRST PRIMARY SITE - STOMACH

| Subsequent primary site | Both tumors microscopically confirmed | | Only 1st tumor microscopically confirmed | | Only 2nd tumor microscopically confirmed | | Neither tumor microscopically confirmed | |
|---|---|---|---|---|---|---|---|---|
| | No. | % | No. | % | No. | % | No. | % |
| SOFT TISSUE | 3 | 100.0 | 0 | 0.0 | 0 | 0.0 | 0 | 0.0 |

Table 29. Subsequent multiple primary malignancies in patients with an index malignant tumor of the small intestine

FIRST PRIMARY SITE - SMALL INTESTINE

| SUBSEQUENT PRIMARY SITES | TOTAL | | | MALES | | | FEMALES | | |
|---|---|---|---|---|---|---|---|---|---|
| | NUMBER OF PERSONS= 362 PERSON-YRS OF OBSERVATION = 942.6 | | | NUMBER OF PERSONS= 190 PERSON-YRS OF OBSERVATION = 504.7 | | | NUMBER OF PERSONS= 172 PERSON-YRS OF OBSERVATION = 437.8 | | |
| | OBS | EXP | OBS/EXP | OBS | EXP | OBS/EXP | OBS | EXP | OBS/EXP |
| LIP | 0 | 0.08 | 0.0 | 0 | 0.08 | 0.0 | 0 | 0.00 | 0.0 |
| TONGUE | 0 | 0.08 | 0.0 | 0 | 0.07 | 0.0 | 0 | 0.01 | 0.0 |
| SALIVARY GLAND | 0 | 0.02 | 0.0 | 0 | 0.02 | 0.0 | 0 | 0.01 | 0.0 |
| MOUTH | 0 | 0.10 | 0.0 | 0 | 0.08 | 0.0 | 0 | 0.02 | 0.0 |
| PHARYNX | 1 | 0.10 | 10.14 | 1 | 0.08 | 11.81 | 0 | 0.01 | 0.0 |
| ESOPHAGUS | 0 | 0.17 | 0.0 | 0 | 0.15 | 0.0 | 0 | 0.02 | 0.0 |
| STOMACH | 1 | 0.71 | 1.41 | 1 | 0.47 | 2.13 | 0 | 0.24 | 0.0 |
| SMALL INTESTINE | 1 | 0.03 | 30.94 | 1 | 0.02 | 55.19* | 0 | 0.01 | 0.0 |
| COLON | 0 | 1.13 | 0.0 | 0 | 0.58 | 0.0 | 0 | 0.55 | 0.0 |
| RECTUM | 0 | 0.60 | 0.0 | 0 | 0.38 | 0.0 | 0 | 0.23 | 0.0 |
| LIVER & BILIARY PASS | 2 | 0.22 | 9.26* | 0 | 0.10 | 0.0 | 2 | 0.11 | 18.02* |
| PANCREAS | 2 | 0.31 | 6.35 | 2 | 0.19 | 10.38* | 0 | 0.12 | 0.0 |
| NOSE AND SINUSES | 0 | 0.02 | 0.0 | 0 | 0.01 | 0.0 | 0 | 0.01 | 0.0 |
| LARYNX | 0 | 0.13 | 0.0 | 0 | 0.13 | 0.0 | 0 | 0.01 | 0.0 |
| LUNG AND BRONCHUS | 1 | 0.85 | 1.18 | 1 | 0.75 | 1.33 | 0 | 0.10 | 0.0 |
| OTHER RESP | 0 | 0.01 | 0.0 | 0 | 0.01 | 0.0 | 0 | 0.00 | 0.0 |
| BREAST | 1 | 0.85 | 1.18 | 0 | 0.01 | 0.0 | 1 | 0.84 | 1.19 |
| CERVIX UTERI | 0 | 0.20 | 0.0 | 0 | 0.0 | 0.0 | 0 | 0.20 | 0.0 |
| CORPUS UTERI | 0 | 0.19 | 0.0 | 0 | 0.0 | 0.0 | 0 | 0.19 | 0.0 |
| UTERUS,UNSPEC | 0 | 0.09 | 0.0 | 0 | 0.0 | 0.0 | 0 | 0.09 | 0.0 |
| OVARY | 3 | 0.17 | 18.12** | 0 | 0.0 | 0.0 | 3 | 0.17 | 18.12** |
| OTHER FEMALE GENITAL | 0 | 0.04 | 0.0 | 0 | 0.0 | 0.0 | 0 | 0.04 | 0.0 |
| PROSTATE | 2 | 0.85 | 2.34 | 2 | 0.85 | 2.34 | 0 | 0.0 | 0.0 |
| TESTIS | 0 | 0.01 | 0.0 | 0 | 0.01 | 0.0 | 0 | 0.0 | 0.0 |
| OTHER MALE GENITAL | 0 | 0.02 | 0.0 | 0 | 0.02 | 0.0 | 0 | 0.0 | 0.0 |
| KIDNEY AND URETER | 0 | 0.18 | 0.0 | 0 | 0.12 | 0.0 | 0 | 0.06 | 0.0 |
| BLADDER | 1 | 0.49 | 2.05 | 0 | 0.38 | 0.0 | 1 | 0.11 | 8.83 |
| MELANOMA OF SKIN | 1 | 0.06 | 16.95 | 1 | 0.03 | 33.74 | 0 | 0.03 | 0.0 |
| EYE | 0 | 0.02 | 0.0 | 0 | 0.01 | 0.0 | 0 | 0.01 | 0.0 |
| NERVOUS SYSTEM | 0 | 0.08 | 0.0 | 0 | 0.05 | 0.0 | 0 | 0.03 | 0.0 |
| THYROID | 0 | 0.04 | 0.0 | 0 | 0.02 | 0.0 | 0 | 0.03 | 0.0 |
| BONE | 0 | 0.02 | 0.0 | 0 | 0.01 | 0.0 | 0 | 0.01 | 0.0 |
| SOFT TISSUE | 0 | 0.06 | 0.0 | 0 | 0.04 | 0.0 | 0 | 0.02 | 0.0 |
| LYMPHOMAS & MYELOMA | 0 | 0.24 | 0.0 | 0 | 0.14 | 0.0 | 0 | 0.10 | 0.0 |
| LEUKEMIAS | 2 | 0.25 | 8.00 | 1 | 0.16 | 6.37 | 1 | 0.09 | 10.77 |
| OTHER SITES | 0 | 0.50 | 0.0 | 0 | 0.28 | 0.0 | 0 | 0.22 | 0.0 |
| TOTAL | 18 | 8.94 | 2.01** | 10 | 5.24 | 1.91 | 8 | 3.69 | 2.17 |

Table 30. Subsequent primary sites with excesses

FIRST PRIMARY SITE - SMALL INTESTINE

| SUBSEQUENT PRIMARY SITES | TOTAL | | | YEARS < 1 | | | YEARS 1-5 | | | YEARS > 5 | | |
|---|---|---|---|---|---|---|---|---|---|---|---|---|
| | NUMBER OF PERSONS= 362 PERSON-YRS OF OBSERVATION= 942.6 | | | NUMBER OF PERSONS= 362 PERSON-YRS OF OBSERVATION= 245.0 | | | NUMBER OF PERSONS= 182 PERSON-YRS OF OBSERVATION= 402.0 | | | NUMBER OF PERSONS= 56 PERSON-YRS OF OBSERVATION= 295.6 | | |
| | OBS | EXP | OBS/EXP | OBS | EXP | OBS/EXP | OBS | EXP | OBS/EXP | OBS | EXP | OBS/EXP |
| SMALL INTESTINE | 1 | 0.03 | 30.94 | 0 | 0.01 | 0.0 | 1 | 0.01 | 73.12* | 0 | 0.01 | 0.0 |
| LIVER & BILIARY PASS | 2 | 0.22 | 9.26* | 1 | 0.05 | 20.15 | 0 | 0.09 | 0.0 | 1 | 0.08 | 12.90 |
| PANCREAS | 2 | 0.31 | 6.35 | 1 | 0.07 | 14.59 | 1 | 0.13 | 7.86 | 0 | 0.12 | 0.0 |
| OVARY | 3 | 0.17 | 18.12** | 2 | 0.04 | 48.46** | 0 | 0.07 | 0.0 | 1 | 0.05 | 19.59 |
| MELANOMA OF SKIN | 1 | 0.06 | 16.95 | 0 | 0.01 | 0.0 | 0 | 0.02 | 0.0 | 1 | 0.02 | 48.34* |
| LEUKEMIAS | 2 | 0.25 | 8.00 | 0 | 0.05 | 0.0 | 0 | 0.10 | 0.0 | 2 | 0.09 | 21.06** |

Table 31. Histologic confirmation of multiple primary malignancies

FIRST PRIMARY SITE - SMALL INTESTINE

| Subsequent primary site | Both tumors microscopically confirmed | | Only 1st tumor microscopically confirmed | | Only 2nd tumor microscopically confirmed | | Neither tumor microscopically confirmed | |
|---|---|---|---|---|---|---|---|---|
| | No. | % | No. | % | No. | % | No. | % |
| SMALL INTESTINE | 1 | 100.0 | 0 | 0.0 | 0 | 0.0 | 0 | 0.0 |
| LIVER & BILIARY PASS | 2 | 100.0 | 0 | 0.0 | 0 | 0.0 | 0 | 0.0 |
| PANCREAS | 2 | 100.0 | 0 | 0.0 | 0 | 0.0 | 0 | 0.0 |
| OVARY | 2 | 66.7 | 0 | 0.0 | 1 | 33.3 | 0 | 0.0 |
| MELANOMA OF SKIN | 1 | 100.0 | 0 | 0.0 | 0 | 0.0 | 0 | 0.0 |
| LEUKEMIAS | 2 | 100.0 | 0 | 0.0 | 0 | 0.0 | 0 | 0.0 |

Table 32. Subsequent multiple primary malignancies in patients with an index malignant tumor of the colon

FIRST PRIMARY SITE - COLON

| | TOTAL | | | MALES | | | FEMALES | | |
|---|---|---|---|---|---|---|---|---|---|
| | NUMBER OF PERSONS= 12729 PERSON-YRS OF OBSERVATION = 42299.4 | | | NUMBER OF PERSONS= 5814 PERSON-YRS OF OBSERVATION = 17790.2 | | | NUMBER OF PERSONS= 6915 PERSON-YRS OF OBSERVATION = 24509.2 | | |
| SUBSEQUENT PRIMARY SITES | OBS | EXP | OBS/EXP | OBS | EXP | OBS/EXP | OBS | EXP | OBS/EXP |
| LIP | 3 | 3.90 | 0.77 | 3 | 3.59 | 0.84 | 0 | 0.31 | 0.0 |
| TONGUE | 2 | 3.59 | 0.56 | 2 | 2.98 | 0.67 | 0 | 0.61 | 0.0 |
| SALIVARY GLAND | 1 | 1.34 | 0.75 | 1 | 0.69 | 1.45 | 0 | 0.65 | 0.0 |
| MOUTH | 7 | 4.83 | 1.45 | 2 | 3.72 | 0.54 | 5 | 1.11 | 4.51* |
| PHARYNX | 5 | 4.53 | 1.10 | 3 | 3.70 | 0.81 | 2 | 0.83 | 2.40 |
| ESOPHAGUS | 11 | 8.05 | 1.37 | 8 | 6.71 | 1.19 | 3 | 1.34 | 2.24 |
| STOMACH | 34 | 38.89 | 0.87 | 23 | 22.94 | 1.00 | 11 | 15.96 | 0.69 |
| SMALL INTESTINE | 9 | 1.70 | 5.31** | 3 | 0.79 | 3.80 | 6 | 0.91 | 6.63** |
| COLON | 134 | 63.59 | 2.11** | 58 | 28.17 | 2.06** | 76 | 35.42 | 2.15** |
| RECTUM | 61 | 32.21 | 1.89** | 31 | 17.62 | 1.76** | 30 | 14.59 | 2.06** |
| LIVER & BILIARY PASS | 14 | 12.51 | 1.12 | 5 | 5.06 | 0.99 | 9 | 7.45 | 1.21 |
| PANCREAS | 13 | 17.02 | 0.76 | 4 | 9.26 | 0.43 | 9 | 7.76 | 1.16 |
| NOSE AND SINUSES | 3 | 0.92 | 3.26 | 1 | 0.54 | 1.86 | 2 | 0.38 | 5.23 |
| LARYNX | 4 | 5.77 | 0.69 | 4 | 5.35 | 0.75 | 0 | 0.42 | 0.0 |
| LUNG AND BRONCHUS | 36 | 37.22 | 0.97 | 30 | 31.13 | 0.96 | 6 | 6.09 | 0.98 |
| OTHER RESP | 2 | 0.63 | 3.20 | 1 | 0.46 | 2.16 | 1 | 0.16 | 6.20 |
| BREAST | 57 | 52.75 | 1.08 | 2 | 0.58 | 3.42 | 55 | 52.17 | 1.05 |
| CERVIX UTERI | 14 | 11.07 | 1.27 | 0 | 0.0 | 0.0 | 14 | 11.07 | 1.27 |
| CORPUS UTERI | 32 | 11.17 | 2.86** | 0 | 0.0 | 0.0 | 32 | 11.17 | 2.86** |
| UTERUS,UNSPEC | 10 | 5.96 | 1.68 | 0 | 0.0 | 0.0 | 10 | 5.96 | 1.68 |
| OVARY | 47 | 9.97 | 4.71** | 0 | 0.0 | 0.0 | 47 | 9.97 | 4.71** |
| OTHER FEMALE GENITAL | 5 | 2.56 | 1.95 | 0 | 0.0 | 0.0 | 5 | 2.56 | 1.95 |
| PROSTATE | 73 | 46.14 | 1.58** | 73 | 46.14 | 1.58** | 0 | 0.0 | 0.0 |
| TESTIS | 1 | 0.43 | 2.31 | 1 | 0.43 | 2.31 | 0 | 0.0 | 0.0 |
| OTHER MALE GENITAL | 0 | 0.85 | 0.0 | 0 | 0.85 | 0.0 | 0 | 0.0 | 0.0 |
| KIDNEY AND URETER | 15 | 8.83 | 1.70 | 11 | 5.28 | 2.09* | 4 | 3.55 | 1.13 |
| BLADDER | 35 | 25.09 | 1.39* | 21 | 17.81 | 1.18 | 14 | 7.28 | 1.92* |
| MELANOMA OF SKIN | 6 | 2.94 | 2.04 | 2 | 1.28 | 1.56 | 4 | 1.65 | 2.42 |
| EYE | 2 | 0.88 | 2.29 | 1 | 0.41 | 2.45 | 1 | 0.47 | 2.14 |
| NERVOUS SYSTEM | 5 | 3.57 | 1.40 | 2 | 1.64 | 1.22 | 3 | 1.93 | 1.56 |
| THYROID | 3 | 2.32 | 1.29 | 2 | 0.64 | 3.12 | 1 | 1.68 | 0.59 |
| BONE | 2 | 1.18 | 1.69 | 1 | 0.55 | 1.80 | 1 | 0.63 | 1.59 |
| SOFT TISSUE | 6 | 2.95 | 2.04 | 3 | 1.54 | 1.95 | 3 | 1.40 | 2.14 |
| LYMPHOMAS & MYELOMA | 9 | 12.39 | 0.73 | 3 | 6.26 | 0.48 | 6 | 6.14 | 0.98 |
| LEUKEMIAS | 10 | 13.04 | 0.77 | 7 | 7.28 | 0.96 | 3 | 5.75 | 0.52 |
| OTHER SITES | 12 | 27.59 | 0.43** | 8 | 13.21 | 0.61 | 4 | 14.37 | 0.28** |
| TOTAL | 683 | 478.36 | 1.43** | 316 | 246.62 | 1.28** | 367 | 231.74 | 1.58** |

Table 33. Subsequent primary sites with excesses

FIRST PRIMARY SITE - COLON

| SUBSEQUENT PRIMARY SITES | TOTAL | | | YEARS < 1 | | | YEARS 1-5 | | | YEARS > 5 | | |
|---|---|---|---|---|---|---|---|---|---|---|---|---|
| | NUMBER OF PERSONS= 12729 PERSON-YRS OF OBSERVATION= 42299.4 | | | NUMBER OF PERSONS= 12729 PERSON-YRS OF OBSERVATION= 9261.3 | | | NUMBER OF PERSONS= 7275 PERSON-YRS OF OBSERVATION= 17625.8 | | | NUMBER OF PERSONS= 2807 PERSON-YRS OF OBSERVATION= 15412.2 | | |
| | OBS | EXP | OBS/EXP | OBS | EXP | OBS/EXP | OBS | EXP | OBS/EXP | OBS | EXP | OBS/EXP |
| MOUTH | 7 | 4.83 | 1.45 | 1 | 1.02 | 0.98 | 0 | 1.97 | 0.0 | 6 | 1.84 | 3.26* |
| SMALL INTESTINE | 9 | 1.70 | 5.31** | 2 | 0.34 | 5.87 | 5 | 0.68 | 7.40** | 2 | 0.68 | 2.94 |
| COLON | 134 | 63.59 | 2.11** | 22 | 12.48 | 1.76* | 61 | 25.13 | 2.43** | 51 | 25.98 | 1.96** |
| RECTUM | 61 | 32.21 | 1.89** | 11 | 6.58 | 1.67 | 29 | 13.02 | 2.23** | 21 | 12.62 | 1.66* |
| CORPUS UTERI | 32 | 11.17 | 2.86** | 5 | 2.14 | 2.33 | 13 | 4.43 | 2.94** | 14 | 4.60 | 3.05** |
| OVARY | 47 | 9.97 | 4.71** | 13 | 1.98 | 6.55** | 28 | 4.00 | 7.00** | 6 | 3.99 | 1.50 |
| PROSTATE | 73 | 46.14 | 1.58** | 19 | 9.23 | 2.06** | 25 | 18.66 | 1.34 | 29 | 18.25 | 1.59* |
| KIDNEY AND URETER | 15 | 8.83 | 1.70 | 6 | 1.78 | 3.36* | 5 | 3.57 | 1.40 | 4 | 3.47 | 1.15 |
| BLADDER | 35 | 25.09 | 1.39* | 8 | 5.02 | 1.59 | 16 | 10.05 | 1.59 | 11 | 10.02 | 1.10 |

Table 34. Subsequent primary sites with deficiencies

FIRST PRIMARY SITE - COLON

| SUBSEQUENT PRIMARY SITES | TOTAL | | | YEARS < 1 | | | YEARS 1-5 | | | YEARS > 5 | | |
|---|---|---|---|---|---|---|---|---|---|---|---|---|
| | NUMBER OF PERSONS= 12729 PERSON-YRS OF OBSERVATION= 42299.4 | | | NUMBER OF PERSONS= 12729 PERSON-YRS OF OBSERVATION= 9261.3 | | | NUMBER OF PERSONS= 7275 PERSON-YRS OF OBSERVATION= 17625.8 | | | NUMBER OF PERSONS= 2807 PERSON-YRS OF OBSERVATION= 15412.2 | | |
| | OBS | EXP | OBS/EXP | OBS | EXP | OBS/EXP | OBS | EXP | OBS/EXP | OBS | EXP | OBS/EXP |
| OTHER SITES | 12 | 27.59 | 0.43** | 0 | 5.31 | 0.0 | 3 | 10.81 | 0.28* | 9 | 11.47 | 0.78 |

Table 35. Histologic confirmation of multiple primary malignancies

FIRST PRIMARY SITE - COLON

| Subsequent primary site | Both tumors microscopically confirmed | | Only 1st tumor microscopically confirmed | | Only 2nd tumor microscopically confirmed | | Neither tumor microscopically confirmed | |
|---|---|---|---|---|---|---|---|---|
| | No. | % | No. | % | No. | % | No. | % |
| MOUTH | 7 | 100.0 | 0 | 0.0 | 0 | 0.0 | 0 | 0.0 |
| SMALL INTESTINE | 9 | 100.0 | 0 | 0.0 | 0 | 0.0 | 0 | 0.0 |
| COLON | 117 | 87.3 | 10 | 7.5 | 5 | 3.7 | 2 | 1.5 |
| RECTUM | 56 | 91.8 | 2 | 3.3 | 3 | 4.9 | 0 | 0.0 |
| CORPUS UTERI | 29 | 90.6 | 0 | 0.0 | 1 | 3.1 | 2 | 6.3 |
| OVARY | 44 | 93.6 | 2 | 4.3 | 1 | 2.1 | 0 | 0.0 |
| PROSTATE | 58 | 79.5 | 11 | 15.1 | 2 | 2.7 | 2 | 2.7 |
| KIDNEY AND URETER | 13 | 86.7 | 0 | 0.0 | 2 | 13.3 | 0 | 0.0 |
| BLADDER | 30 | 85.7 | 4 | 11.4 | 1 | 2.9 | 0 | 0.0 |

Table 36. Subsequent multiple primary malignancies in patients with an index malignant tumor of the rectum

FIRST PRIMARY SITE - RECTUM

| SUBSEQUENT PRIMARY SITES | TOTAL | | | MALES | | | FEMALES | | |
|---|---|---|---|---|---|---|---|---|---|
| | NUMBER OF PERSONS= 8083 PERSON-YRS OF OBSERVATION = 26059.9 | | | NUMBER OF PERSONS= 4533 PERSON-YRS OF OBSERVATION = 13478.2 | | | NUMBER OF PERSONS= 3550 PERSON-YRS OF OBSERVATION = 12581.7 | | |
| | OBS | EXP | OBS/EXP | OBS | EXP | OBS/EXP | OBS | EXP | OBS/EXP |
| LIP | 1 | 2.73 | 0.37 | 1 | 2.58 | 0.39 | 0 | 0.15 | 0.0 |
| TONGUE | 3 | 2.43 | 1.24 | 3 | 2.13 | 1.41 | 0 | 0.30 | 0.0 |
| SALIVARY GLAND | 1 | 0.80 | 1.26 | 1 | 0.48 | 2.07 | 0 | 0.31 | 0.0 |
| MOUTH | 4 | 3.17 | 1.26 | 3 | 2.65 | 1.13 | 1 | 0.52 | 1.92 |
| PHARYNX | 1 | 3.09 | 0.32 | 1 | 2.67 | 0.37 | 0 | 0.42 | 0.0 |
| ESOPHAGUS | 3 | 5.50 | 0.55 | 3 | 4.85 | 0.62 | 0 | 0.65 | 0.0 |
| STOMACH | 7 | 23.83 | 0.29** | 6 | 16.24 | 0.37** | 1 | 7.59 | 0.13** |
| SMALL INTESTINE | 2 | 0.99 | 2.01 | 1 | 0.56 | 1.77 | 1 | 0.43 | 2.33 |
| COLON | 61 | 36.11 | 1.69** | 36 | 19.33 | 1.86** | 25 | 16.78 | 1.49 |
| RECTUM | 4 | 19.50 | 0.21** | 1 | 12.44 | 0.08** | 3 | 7.06 | 0.42 |
| LIVER & BILIARY PASS | 4 | 7.11 | 0.56 | 3 | 3.56 | 0.84 | 1 | 3.55 | 0.28 |
| PANCREAS | 2 | 10.03 | 0.20** | 1 | 6.36 | 0.16* | 1 | 3.67 | 0.27 |
| NOSE AND SINUSES | 1 | 0.56 | 1.79 | 0 | 0.37 | 0.0 | 1 | 0.18 | 5.44 |
| LARYNX | 6 | 4.07 | 1.47 | 6 | 3.86 | 1.55 | 0 | 0.21 | 0.0 |
| LUNG AND BRONCHUS | 13 | 25.14 | 0.52* | 11 | 22.23 | 0.49* | 2 | 2.91 | 0.69 |
| OTHER RESP | 0 | 0.41 | 0.0 | 0 | 0.33 | 0.0 | 0 | 0.08 | 0.0 |
| BREAST | 27 | 26.14 | 1.03 | 0 | 0.41 | 0.0 | 27 | 25.73 | 1.05 |
| CERVIX UTERI | 4 | 5.76 | 0.69 | 0 | 0.0 | 0.0 | 4 | 5.76 | 0.69 |
| CORPUS UTERI | 9 | 5.60 | 1.61 | 0 | 0.0 | 0.0 | 9 | 5.60 | 1.61 |
| UTERUS,UNSPEC | 1 | 3.03 | 0.33 | 0 | 0.0 | 0.0 | 1 | 3.03 | 0.33 |
| OVARY | 11 | 5.03 | 2.19* | 0 | 0.0 | 0.0 | 11 | 5.03 | 2.19* |
| OTHER FEMALE GENITAL | 1 | 1.21 | 0.83 | 0 | 0.0 | 0.0 | 1 | 1.21 | 0.83 |
| PROSTATE | 55 | 30.11 | 1.83** | 55 | 30.11 | 1.83** | 0 | 0.0 | 0.0 |
| TESTIS | 1 | 0.32 | 3.14 | 1 | 0.32 | 3.14 | 0 | 0.0 | 0.0 |
| OTHER MALE GENITAL | 0 | 0.61 | 0.0 | 0 | 0.61 | 0.0 | 0 | 0.0 | 0.0 |
| KIDNEY AND URETER | 3 | 5.43 | 0.55 | 3 | 3.72 | 0.81 | 0 | 1.70 | 0.0 |
| BLADDER | 20 | 15.60 | 1.28 | 19 | 12.22 | 1.55 | 1 | 3.38 | 0.30 |
| MELANOMA OF SKIN | 1 | 1.72 | 0.58 | 1 | 0.90 | 1.11 | 0 | 0.82 | 0.0 |
| EYE | 1 | 0.53 | 1.89 | 0 | 0.30 | 0.0 | 1 | 0.23 | 4.38 |
| NERVOUS SYSTEM | 2 | 2.33 | 0.86 | 2 | 1.32 | 1.52 | 0 | 1.01 | 0.0 |
| THYROID | 0 | 1.26 | 0.0 | 0 | 0.46 | 0.0 | 0 | 0.80 | 0.0 |
| BONE | 1 | 0.71 | 1.40 | 1 | 0.40 | 2.48 | 0 | 0.31 | 0.0 |
| SOFT TISSUE | 2 | 1.75 | 1.15 | 1 | 1.06 | 0.94 | 1 | 0.69 | 1.46 |
| LYMPHOMAS & MYELOMA | 4 | 7.34 | 0.55 | 4 | 4.38 | 0.91 | 0 | 2.96 | 0.0 |
| LEUKEMIAS | 7 | 7.74 | 0.90 | 6 | 5.00 | 1.20 | 1 | 2.74 | 0.37 |
| OTHER SITES | 3 | 15.80 | 0.19** | 2 | 9.06 | 0.22* | 1 | 6.74 | 0.15* |
| TOTAL | 266 | 283.49 | 0.94 | 172 | 170.93 | 1.01 | 94 | 112.56 | 0.84 |

Table 37. Subsequent primary sites with excesses

FIRST PRIMARY SITE - RECTUM

| SUBSEQUENT PRIMARY SITES | TOTAL<br>NUMBER OF PERSONS= 8083<br>PERSON-YRS OF OBSERVATION= 26059.9 | | | YEARS < 1<br>NUMBER OF PERSONS= 8083<br>PERSON-YRS OF OBSERVATION= 6110.8 | | | YEARS 1-5<br>NUMBER OF PERSONS= 4816<br>PERSON-YRS OF OBSERVATION= 11099.0 | | | YEARS > 5<br>NUMBER OF PERSONS= 1658<br>PERSON-YRS OF OBSERVATION= 8850.1 | | |
|---|---|---|---|---|---|---|---|---|---|---|---|---|
| | OBS | EXP | OBS/EXP | OBS | EXP | OBS/EXP | OBS | EXP | OBS/EXP | OBS | EXP | OBS/EXP |
| COLON | 61 | 36.11 | 1.69** | 15 | 7.45 | 2.01* | 18 | 14.38 | 1.25 | 28 | 14.28 | 1.96** |
| OVARY | 11 | 5.03 | 2.19* | 5 | 1.04 | 4.80** | 6 | 2.04 | 2.93* | 0 | 1.94 | 0.0 |
| PROSTATE | 55 | 30.11 | 1.83** | 13 | 6.30 | 2.06* | 21 | 11.83 | 1.78* | 21 | 11.98 | 1.75* |

Table 38. Subsequent primary sites with deficiencies

FIRST PRIMARY SITE - RECTUM

| SUBSEQUENT PRIMARY SITES | TOTAL<br>NUMBER OF PERSONS= 8083<br>PERSON-YRS OF OBSERVATION= 26059.9 | | | YEARS < 1<br>NUMBER OF PERSONS= 8083<br>PERSON-YRS OF OBSERVATION= 6110.8 | | | YEARS 1-5<br>NUMBER OF PERSONS= 4816<br>PERSON-YRS OF OBSERVATION= 11099.0 | | | YEARS > 5<br>NUMBER OF PERSONS= 1658<br>PERSON-YRS OF OBSERVATION= 8850.1 | | |
|---|---|---|---|---|---|---|---|---|---|---|---|---|
| | OBS | EXP | OBS/EXP | OBS | EXP | OBS/EXP | OBS | EXP | OBS/EXP | OBS | EXP | OBS/EXP |
| STOMACH | 7 | 23.83 | 0.29** | 1 | 5.43 | 0.18 | 4 | 9.73 | 0.41 | 2 | 8.66 | 0.23* |
| RECTUM | 4 | 19.50 | 0.21** | 3 | 4.27 | 0.70 | 0 | 7.97 | 0.0 | 1 | 7.26 | 0.14* |
| PANCREAS | 2 | 10.03 | 0.20** | 0 | 2.08 | 0.0 | 1 | 4.00 | 0.25 | 1 | 3.95 | 0.25 |
| LUNG AND BRONCHUS | 13 | 25.14 | 0.52* | 0 | 5.25 | 0.0 | 6 | 10.35 | 0.58 | 7 | 9.53 | 0.73 |
| OTHER SITES | 3 | 15.80 | 0.19** | 0 | 3.18 | 0.0 | 1 | 6.26 | 0.16* | 2 | 6.36 | 0.31 |

Table 39. Histologic confirmation of multiple primary malignancies

FIRST PRIMARY SITE - RECTUM

| Subsequent primary site | Both tumors microscopically confirmed | | Only 1st tumor microscopically confirmed | | Only 2nd tumor microscopically confirmed | | Neither tumor microscopically confirmed | |
|---|---|---|---|---|---|---|---|---|
| | No. | % | No. | % | No. | % | No. | % |
| COLON | 56 | 91.8 | 4 | 6.6 | 1 | 1.6 | 0 | 0.0 |
| OVARY | 10 | 90.9 | 1 | 9.1 | 0 | 0.0 | 0 | 0.0 |
| PROSTATE | 42 | 76.4 | 11 | 20.0 | 2 | 3.6 | 0 | 0.0 |

Table 40. Subsequent multiple primary malignancies in patients with an index malignant tumor of the liver and biliary passages

FIRST PRIMARY SITE - LIVER AND BILIARY PASSAGES

| SUBSEQUENT PRIMARY SITES | TOTAL | | | MALES | | | FEMALES | | |
|---|---|---|---|---|---|---|---|---|---|
| | NUMBER OF PERSONS= 1883 PERSON-YRS OF OBSERVATION = 1253.2 | | | NUMBER OF PERSONS= 777 PERSON-YRS OF OBSERVATION = 437.5 | | | NUMBER OF PERSONS= 1106 PERSON-YRS OF OBSERVATION = 815.7 | | |
| | OBS | EXP | OBS/EXP | OBS | EXP | OBS/EXP | OBS | EXP | OBS/EXP |
| LIP | 0 | 0.09 | 0.0 | 0 | 0.08 | 0.0 | 0 | 0.01 | 0.0 |
| TONGUE | 0 | 0.09 | 0.0 | 0 | 0.07 | 0.0 | 0 | 0.02 | 0.0 |
| SALIVARY GLAND | 0 | 0.04 | 0.0 | 0 | 0.02 | 0.0 | 0 | 0.02 | 0.0 |
| MOUTH | 0 | 0.12 | 0.0 | 0 | 0.08 | 0.0 | 0 | 0.04 | 0.0 |
| PHARYNX | 0 | 0.11 | 0.0 | 0 | 0.08 | 0.0 | 0 | 0.03 | 0.0 |
| ESOPHAGUS | 0 | 0.20 | 0.0 | 0 | 0.15 | 0.0 | 0 | 0.05 | 0.0 |
| STOMACH | 1 | 1.02 | 0.98 | 1 | 0.50 | 2.01 | 0 | 0.52 | 0.0 |
| SMALL INTESTINE | 0 | 0.05 | 0.0 | 0 | 0.02 | 0.0 | 0 | 0.03 | 0.0 |
| COLON | 3 | 1.73 | 1.74 | 1 | 0.59 | 1.68 | 2 | 1.13 | 1.77 |
| RECTUM | 2 | 0.86 | 2.32 | 0 | 0.38 | 0.0 | 2 | 0.48 | 4.17 |
| LIVER & BILIARY PASS | 0 | 0.36 | 0.0 | 0 | 0.11 | 0.0 | 0 | 0.25 | 0.0 |
| PANCREAS | 0 | 0.45 | 0.0 | 0 | 0.20 | 0.0 | 0 | 0.25 | 0.0 |
| NOSE AND SINUSES | 0 | 0.02 | 0.0 | 0 | 0.01 | 0.0 | 0 | 0.01 | 0.0 |
| LARYNX | 0 | 0.14 | 0.0 | 0 | 0.12 | 0.0 | 0 | 0.01 | 0.0 |
| LUNG AND BRONCHUS | 2 | 0.92 | 2.18 | 1 | 0.72 | 1.39 | 1 | 0.20 | 5.09 |
| OTHER RESP | 0 | 0.02 | 0.0 | 0 | 0.01 | 0.0 | 0 | 0.01 | 0.0 |
| BREAST | 1 | 1.72 | 0.58 | 0 | 0.01 | 0.0 | 1 | 1.71 | 0.59 |
| CERVIX UTERI | 1 | 0.37 | 2.71 | 0 | 0.0 | 0.0 | 1 | 0.37 | 2.71 |
| CORPUS UTERI | 0 | 0.38 | 0.0 | 0 | 0.0 | 0.0 | 0 | 0.38 | 0.0 |
| UTERUS,UNSPEC | 0 | 0.21 | 0.0 | 0 | 0.0 | 0.0 | 0 | 0.21 | 0.0 |
| OVARY | 0 | 0.34 | 0.0 | 0 | 0.0 | 0.0 | 0 | 0.34 | 0.0 |
| OTHER FEMALE GENITAL | 0 | 0.08 | 0.0 | 0 | 0.0 | 0.0 | 0 | 0.08 | 0.0 |
| PROSTATE | 5 | 0.89 | 5.59** | 5 | 0.89 | 5.59** | 0 | 0.0 | 0.0 |
| TESTIS | 0 | 0.01 | 0.0 | 0 | 0.01 | 0.0 | 0 | 0.0 | 0.0 |
| OTHER MALE GENITAL | 0 | 0.02 | 0.0 | 0 | 0.02 | 0.0 | 0 | 0.0 | 0.0 |
| KIDNEY AND URETER | 2 | 0.23 | 8.60* | 2 | 0.12 | 17.14* | 0 | 0.12 | 0.0 |
| BLADDER | 0 | 0.60 | 0.0 | 0 | 0.37 | 0.0 | 0 | 0.23 | 0.0 |
| MELANOMA OF SKIN | 0 | 0.08 | 0.0 | 0 | 0.03 | 0.0 | 0 | 0.05 | 0.0 |
| EYE | 0 | 0.02 | 0.0 | 0 | 0.01 | 0.0 | 0 | 0.02 | 0.0 |
| NERVOUS SYSTEM | 0 | 0.11 | 0.0 | 0 | 0.04 | 0.0 | 0 | 0.07 | 0.0 |
| THYROID | 0 | 0.07 | 0.0 | 0 | 0.01 | 0.0 | 0 | 0.05 | 0.0 |
| BONE | 0 | 0.03 | 0.0 | 0 | 0.01 | 0.0 | 0 | 0.02 | 0.0 |
| SOFT TISSUE | 0 | 0.08 | 0.0 | 0 | 0.03 | 0.0 | 0 | 0.04 | 0.0 |
| LYMPHOMAS & MYELOMA | 1 | 0.34 | 2.94 | 1 | 0.14 | 7.21 | 0 | 0.20 | 0.0 |
| LEUKEMIAS | 0 | 0.34 | 0.0 | 0 | 0.15 | 0.0 | 0 | 0.19 | 0.0 |
| OTHER SITES | 0 | 0.74 | 0.0 | 0 | 0.29 | 0.0 | 0 | 0.46 | 0.0 |
| TOTAL | 18 | 12.88 | 1.40 | 11 | 5.30 | 2.08* | 7 | 7.58 | 0.92 |

Table 41. Subsequent primary sites with excesses

FIRST PRIMARY SITE - LIVER AND BILIARY PASSAGES

| SUBSEQUENT PRIMARY SITES | TOTAL | | | YEARS < 1 | | | YEARS 1-5 | | | YEARS > 5 | | |
|---|---|---|---|---|---|---|---|---|---|---|---|---|
| | NUMBER OF PERSONS= 1883 PERSON-YRS OF OBSERVATION= 1253.2 | | | NUMBER OF PERSONS= 1883 PERSON-YRS OF OBSERVATION= 677.7 | | | NUMBER OF PERSONS= 269 PERSON-YRS OF OBSERVATION= 400.7 | | | NUMBER OF PERSONS= 47 PERSON-YRS OF OBSERVATION= 174.8 | | |
| | OBS | EXP | OBS/EXP | OBS | EXP | OBS/EXP | OBS | EXP | OBS/EXP | OBS | EXP | OBS/EXP |
| PROSTATE | 5 | 0.89 | 5.59** | 4 | 0.50 | 7.97** | 1 | 0.26 | 3.91 | 0 | 0.14 | 0.0 |
| KIDNEY AND URETER | 2 | 0.23 | 8.60* | 2 | 0.12 | 16.12* | 0 | 0.07 | 0.0 | 0 | C.03 | 0.0 |

Table 42. Histologic confirmation of multiple primary malignancies

FIRST PRIMARY SITE - LIVER AND BILIARY PASSAGES

| Subsequent primary site | Both tumors microscopically confirmed | | Only 1st tumor microscopically confirmed | | Only 2nd tumor microscopically confirmed | | Neither tumor microscopically confirmed | |
|---|---|---|---|---|---|---|---|---|
| | No. | % | No. | % | No. | % | No. | % |
| PROSTATE | 3 | 60.0 | 1 | 20.0 | 1 | 20.0 | 0 | 0.0 |
| KIDNEY AND URETER | 2 | 100.0 | 0 | 0.0 | 0 | 0.0 | 0 | 0.0 |

Table 43. Subsequent multiple primary malignancies in patients with an index malignant tumor of the pancreas

FIRST PRIMARY SITE - PANCREAS

| SUBSEQUENT PRIMARY SITES | TOTAL NUMBER OF PERSONS= 2670 PERSON-YRS OF OBSERVATION = 1370.9 | | | MALES NUMBER OF PERSONS= 1550 PERSON-YRS OF OBSERVATION = 709.2 | | | FEMALES NUMBER OF PERSONS= 1120 PERSON-YRS OF OBSERVATION = 661.7 | | |
|---|---|---|---|---|---|---|---|---|---|
| | OBS | EXP | OBS/EXP | OBS | EXP | OBS/EXP | OBS | EXP | OBS/EXP |
| LIP | 0 | 0.14 | 0.0 | 0 | 0.13 | 0.0 | 0 | 0.01 | 0.0 |
| TONGUE | 0 | 0.12 | 0.0 | 0 | 0.11 | 0.0 | 0 | 0.02 | 0.0 |
| SALIVARY GLAND | 0 | 0.04 | 0.0 | 0 | 0.02 | 0.0 | 0 | 0.02 | 0.0 |
| MOUTH | 0 | 0.16 | 0.0 | 0 | 0.14 | 0.0 | 0 | 0.03 | 0.0 |
| PHARYNX | 1 | 0.16 | 6.40 | 0 | 0.13 | 0.0 | 1 | 0.02 | 45.66* |
| ESOPHAGUS | 0 | 0.28 | 0.0 | 0 | 0.24 | 0.0 | 0 | 0.04 | 0.0 |
| STOMACH | 0 | 1.24 | 0.0 | 0 | 0.83 | 0.0 | 0 | 0.41 | 0.0 |
| SMALL INTESTINE | 0 | 0.05 | 0.0 | 0 | 0.03 | 0.0 | 0 | 0.02 | 0.0 |
| COLON | 1 | 1.83 | 0.55 | 1 | 0.98 | 1.02 | 0 | 0.86 | 0.0 |
| RECTUM | 0 | 0.99 | 0.0 | 0 | 0.62 | 0.0 | 0 | 0.37 | 0.0 |
| LIVER & BILIARY PASS | 0 | 0.37 | 0.0 | 0 | 0.18 | 0.0 | 0 | 0.19 | 0.0 |
| PANCREAS | 0 | 0.52 | 0.0 | 0 | 0.33 | 0.0 | 0 | 0.19 | 0.0 |
| NOSE AND SINUSES | 0 | 0.03 | 0.0 | 0 | 0.02 | 0.0 | 0 | 0.01 | 0.0 |
| LARYNX | 0 | 0.20 | 0.0 | 0 | 0.19 | 0.0 | 0 | 0.01 | 0.0 |
| LUNG AND BRONCHUS | 0 | 1.24 | 0.0 | 0 | 1.09 | 0.0 | 0 | 0.15 | 0.0 |
| OTHER RESP | 1 | 0.02 | 46.43* | 1 | 0.02 | 58.71* | 0 | 0.00 | 0.0 |
| BREAST | 0 | 1.36 | 0.0 | 0 | 0.02 | 0.0 | 0 | 1.34 | 0.0 |
| CERVIX UTERI | 0 | 0.30 | 0.0 | 0 | 0.0 | 0.0 | 0 | 0.30 | 0.0 |
| CORPUS UTERI | 0 | 0.29 | 0.0 | 0 | 0.0 | 0.0 | 0 | 0.29 | 0.0 |
| UTERUS,UNSPEC | 1 | 0.17 | 6.04 | 0 | 0.0 | 0.0 | 1 | 0.17 | 6.04 |
| OVARY | 0 | 0.26 | 0.0 | 0 | 0.0 | 0.0 | 0 | 0.26 | 0.0 |
| OTHER FEMALE GENITAL | 0 | 0.06 | 0.0 | 0 | 0.0 | 0.0 | 0 | 0.06 | 0.0 |
| PROSTATE | 8 | 1.55 | 5.16** | 8 | 1.55 | 5.16** | 0 | 0.0 | 0.0 |
| TESTIS | 1 | 0.02 | 59.12* | 1 | 0.02 | 59.12* | 0 | 0.0 | 0.0 |
| OTHER MALE GENITAL | 0 | 0.03 | 0.0 | 0 | 0.03 | 0.0 | 0 | 0.0 | 0.0 |
| KIDNEY AND URETER | 0 | 0.27 | 0.0 | 0 | 0.19 | 0.0 | 0 | 0.09 | 0.0 |
| BLADDER | 0 | 0.78 | 0.0 | 0 | 0.61 | 0.0 | 0 | 0.17 | 0.0 |
| MELANOMA OF SKIN | 0 | 0.09 | 0.0 | 0 | 0.05 | 0.0 | 0 | 0.04 | 0.0 |
| EYE | 0 | 0.03 | 0.0 | 0 | 0.01 | 0.0 | 0 | 0.01 | 0.0 |
| NERVOUS SYSTEM | 0 | 0.12 | 0.0 | 0 | 0.07 | 0.0 | 0 | 0.05 | 0.0 |
| THYROID | 1 | 0.06 | 15.84 | 1 | 0.02 | 44.27* | 0 | 0.04 | 0.0 |
| BONE | 0 | 0.04 | 0.0 | 0 | 0.02 | 0.0 | 0 | 0.02 | 0.0 |
| SOFT TISSUE | 0 | 0.09 | 0.0 | 0 | 0.06 | 0.0 | 0 | 0.03 | 0.0 |
| LYMPHOMAS & MYELOMA | 0 | 0.37 | 0.0 | 0 | 0.22 | 0.0 | 0 | 0.15 | 0.0 |
| LEUKEMIAS | 1 | 0.39 | 2.54 | 1 | 0.25 | 3.95 | 0 | 0.14 | 0.0 |
| OTHER SITES | 0 | 0.79 | 0.0 | 0 | 0.46 | 0.0 | 0 | 0.33 | 0.0 |
| TOTAL | 15 | 14.47 | 1.04 | 13 | 8.64 | 1.51 | 2 | 5.83 | 0.34 |

Table 44. Subsequent primary sites with excesses

FIRST PRIMARY SITE - PANCREAS

| SUBSEQUENT PRIMARY SITES | TOTAL | | | YEARS < 1 | | | YEARS 1-5 | | | YEARS > 5 | | |
|---|---|---|---|---|---|---|---|---|---|---|---|---|
| | NUMBER OF PERSONS= 2670 PERSON-YRS OF OBSERVATION= 1370.9 | | | NUMBER OF PERSONS= 2670 PERSON-YRS OF OBSERVATION= 935.9 | | | NUMBER OF PERSONS= 295 PERSON-YRS OF OBSERVATION= 321.3 | | | NUMBER OF PERSONS= 29 PERSON-YRS OF OBSERVATION= 113.7 | | |
| | OBS | EXP | OBS/EXP | OBS | EXP | OBS/EXP | OBS | EXP | OBS/EXP | OBS | EXP | OBS/EXP |
| PHARYNX | 1 | 0.16 | 6.40 | 0 | 0.11 | 0.0 | 1 | 0.04 | 28.14 | 0 | 0.01 | 0.0 |
| OTHER RESP | 1 | 0.02 | 46.43* | 1 | 0.02 | 63.88* | 0 | 0.00 | 0.0 | 0 | 0.00 | 0.0 |
| PROSTATE | 8 | 1.55 | 5.16** | 7 | 1.10 | 6.34** | 1 | 0.41 | 2.45 | 0 | 0.04 | 0.0 |
| TESTIS | 1 | 0.02 | 59.12* | 1 | 0.01 | 81.43* | 0 | 0.00 | 0.0 | 0 | 0.00 | 0.0 |
| THYROID | 1 | 0.06 | 15.84 | 1 | 0.04 | 23.55 | 0 | 0.02 | 0.0 | 0 | 0.01 | 0.0 |

Table 45. Histologic confirmation of multiple primary malignancies

FIRST PRIMARY SITE - PANCREAS

| Subsequent primary site | Both tumors microscopically confirmed | | Only 1st tumor microscopically confirmed | | Only 2nd tumor microscopically confirmed | | Neither tumor microscopically confirmed | |
|---|---|---|---|---|---|---|---|---|
| | No. | % | No. | % | No. | % | No. | % |
| PHARYNX | 0 | 0.0 | 0 | 0.0 | 1 | 100.0 | 0 | 0.0 |
| OTHER RESP | 1 | 100.0 | 0 | 0.0 | 0 | 0.0 | 0 | 0.0 |
| PROSTATE | 7 | 87.5 | 0 | 0.0 | 1 | 12.5 | 0 | 0.0 |
| TESTIS | 1 | 100.0 | 0 | 0.0 | 0 | 0.0 | 0 | 0.0 |
| THYROID | 1 | 100.0 | 0 | 0.0 | 0 | 0.0 | 0 | 0.0 |

Table 46. Summary of site-group pairs with an excess of observed-over-expected subsequent primary malignancies: index tumors of the digestive system

I. Possibly artifact

- Colon → Prostate
- Rectum → Prostate
- Liver/biliary passages → Prostate
- Pancreas → Prostate
- Small intestine → Ovary
- Small intestine → Melanoma (skin)
- Small intestine → Leukemia
- Liver/biliary passages → Kidney/ureter
- Pancreas → Pharynx
- Pancreas → Other respiratory organs
- Pancreas → Testis
- Pancreas → Thyroid

II. Possibly real

A. In organs within the same system

1. Same or paired organs

- Esophagus ↔ Esophagus
- Small intestine ↔ Small intestine
- Colon ↔ Colon

2. Others

- Colon ↔ Rectum
- Small intestine → Liver/biliary passages
- Small intestine → Pancreas
- Colon → Small intestine

B. In organs related structurally or functionally

- Esophagus ↔ Mouth
- Esophagus → Lip
- Esophagus → Larynx
- Colon → Mouth

C. In organs apparently unrelated structurally or functionally

- Colon ↔ Corpus uteri
- Colon ↔ Ovary
- Rectum → Ovary
- Stomach → Soft tissue
- Colon → Kidney/ureter
- Colon → Bladder

Table 47. Summary of site-group pairs with a deficiency of observed-over-expected subsequent primary malignancies: index tumors of the digestive system

I. In the same organ

- Stomach → Stomach
- Rectum → Rectum

II. In different organs

- Rectum → Stomach
- Rectum → Pancreas
- Rectum → Lung/bronchus
- Rectum → Other/unspecified sites
- Colon → Other/unspecified sites

Table 48. Common metastatic sites for primary malignant tumors of the digestive system (HOLLAND and FREI, 1973; WILLIS, 1973; RUBIN, 1974)

| Anatomic location of the primary malignant tumor | Common metastatic sites |
|---|---|
| Esophagus | Liver; lung and pleura; intrathoracic organs; paraesophageal lymph nodes |
| Stomach | Perigastric, left supraclavicular, left anterior axillary, and inguinal lymph nodes; liver; lung; bone; brain; skin and subcutaneous tissues; skeletal muscle; parietal peritoneum (rectal shelf); ovary (Krukenberg tumor) |
| Small intestine | Mesenteric lymph nodes; peritoneum; liver; brain |
| Colon, rectum, and anus | Regional, periaortic, and perineal lymph nodes; liver; stomach; pancreas; kidney; bladder; prostate; duodenum; spleen; brain; ureter; vagina; sacrum and sacral nerves; retroperitoneal area; abdominal wall |
| Liver and biliary passages | Periportal, duodenal, retroperitoneal, and distant lymph nodes; other parts of liver; lung and pleura; stomach; colon; rectum, peritoneum; adrenals; ovaries; brain |
| Pancreas | Peritoneum; lung and pleura; liver; regional lymph nodes; gallbladder; spleen; adrenal glands; intestine; brain and spinal cord; bone |

# Chapter 8

# Index Tumors of the Respiratory System

Population studied. 8,730 males and 1,540 females with cancer of the respiratory system were followed for the subsequent development of independent primary malignant neoplasms; 271 such subsequent neoplasms were diagnosed. The cohort of individuals with cancer of the respiratory system contributed 15,437 person-years of observation.

Results. Detailed tabulations by site are presented in Tables 49-60. The reader is referred to Chapter 5 for a general explanation of the items in these tables.

Summary of Findings. Site-group pairs with a statistically significant excess of observed-over-expected subsequent primary cancers are categorized in Table 61 on the basis of possible relationships between the anatomic sites containing these cancers. In addition, possible artifactual relationships, based on a small number of cases and with no confirmation from other published reports, are emphasized.

Discussion. Table 62 presents the common metastatic sites for cancers arising within the respiratory system. These data, used in conjunction with the site-specific tabulations of the percentage of multiple primary malignancies with histologic confirmation, are useful in distinguishing real from artifactual associations.

The excess risk of prostatic cancer in patients with cancer of the respiratory system is thought to be spurious. Asymptomatic prostatic malignancies which might otherwise go unnoticed, are first diagnosed at autopsy performed on patients dying with respiratory malignancies. The excess of breast cancer among patients with cancer of the nose or sinuses is based on a total of only four observed cases. The remaining relationships listed in category I are based on one or two observed cases. None of these associations are supported by the findings of other studies.

The relationship among cancers of the larynx, lung, and bronchus demonstrated in the Connecticut data (category IIA) is supported by the findings of other studies (CAHAN and MONTEMAYOR, 1962; BERG et al., 1970). Smoking has been suggested as a common etiologic factor. The excess risk of cancer of tongue and pharynx in patients with laryngeal cancer represents another example of the relationship among cancers of the oral cavity, pharynx, respiratory system, and upper digestive system. A detailed analysis of this association is described in Chapter 6. Once again, smoking may be an important common etiologic agent in the pathogenesis of these malignancies.

The site-group pairs noted in category IIC may also be related by a common etiologic agent. Cigarette smokers are at increased risk for cancers of the lung and larynx (HAMMOND, 1966; LEVIN et al., 1974; HAMMOND, 1975). Cancer of the urinary bladder has also been shown to be related to heavy cigarette smoking (LILIENFELD et al., 1956; HAMMOND, 1966; LEVIN et al., 1974; HAMMOND, 1975). Finally, a prospective epidemiologic study of a large cohort found that the risk of dying from kidney cancer was two- to three-times increased for men with a history of cigarette smoking as compared to men who never smoked (HAMMOND, 1975). Other reports have documented the occurrence of lung and kidney cancer in the same patient (MOERTEL, 1966; CAHAN, 1969), but only the present study demonstrates that this association occurs more frequently than might be expected on the basis of chance.

Table 49. Subsequent multiple primary malignancies in patients with an index malignant tumor of the nose and sinuses

FIRST PRIMARY SITE - NOSE,NASAL CAVITIES,MIDDLE EAR,AND ACCESSORY SINUSES

| SUBSEQUENT PRIMARY SITES | TOTAL NUMBER OF PERSONS= 338 PERSON-YRS OF OBSERVATION = 1207.2 | | | MALES NUMBER OF PERSONS= 211 PERSON-YRS OF OBSERVATION = 754.9 | | | FEMALES NUMBER OF PERSONS= 127 PERSON-YRS OF OBSERVATION = 452.2 | | |
|---|---|---|---|---|---|---|---|---|---|
| | OBS | EXP | OBS/EXP | OBS | EXP | OBS/EXP | OBS | EXP | OBS/EXP |
| LIP | 0 | 0.13 | 0.0 | 0 | 0.13 | 0.0 | 0 | 0.01 | 0.0 |
| TONGUE | 1 | 0.11 | 9.11 | 1 | 0.10 | 9.99 | 0 | 0.01 | 0.0 |
| SALIVARY GLAND | 0 | 0.03 | 0.0 | 0 | 0.02 | 0.0 | 0 | 0.01 | 0.0 |
| MOUTH | 0 | 0.14 | 0.0 | 0 | 0.12 | 0.0 | 0 | 0.02 | 0.0 |
| PHARYNX | 0 | 0.14 | 0.0 | 0 | 0.13 | 0.0 | 0 | 0.01 | 0.0 |
| ESOPHAGUS | 0 | 0.25 | 0.0 | 0 | 0.22 | 0.0 | 0 | 0.02 | 0.0 |
| STOMACH | 0 | 1.01 | 0.0 | 0 | 0.76 | 0.0 | 0 | 0.25 | 0.0 |
| SMALL INTESTINE | 0 | 0.04 | 0.0 | 0 | 0.03 | 0.0 | 0 | 0.01 | 0.0 |
| COLON | 3 | 1.40 | 2.15 | 2 | 0.86 | 2.33 | 1 | 0.54 | 1.86 |
| RECTUM | 0 | 0.79 | 0.0 | 0 | 0.57 | 0.0 | 0 | 0.22 | 0.0 |
| LIVER & BILIARY PASS | 0 | 0.28 | 0.0 | 0 | 0.16 | 0.0 | 0 | 0.12 | 0.0 |
| PANCREAS | 0 | 0.40 | 0.0 | 0 | 0.28 | 0.0 | 0 | 0.12 | 0.0 |
| NOSE AND SINUSES | 0 | 0.03 | 0.0 | 0 | 0.02 | 0.0 | 0 | 0.01 | 0.0 |
| LARYNX | 0 | 0.18 | 0.0 | 0 | 0.18 | 0.0 | 0 | 0.01 | 0.0 |
| LUNG AND BRONCHUS | 0 | 1.08 | 0.0 | 0 | 0.98 | 0.0 | 0 | 0.10 | 0.0 |
| OTHER RESP | 0 | 0.02 | 0.0 | 0 | 0.02 | 0.0 | 0 | 0.00 | 0.0 |
| BREAST | 4 | 0.87 | 4.60* | 0 | 0.02 | 0.0 | 4 | 0.85 | 4.70* |
| CERVIX UTERI | 0 | 0.20 | 0.0 | 0 | 0.0 | 0.0 | 0 | 0.20 | 0.0 |
| CORPUS UTERI | 0 | 0.17 | 0.0 | 0 | 0.0 | 0.0 | 0 | 0.17 | 0.0 |
| UTERUS,UNSPEC | 0 | 0.10 | 0.0 | 0 | 0.0 | 0.0 | 0 | 0.10 | 0.0 |
| OVARY | 0 | 0.16 | 0.0 | 0 | 0.0 | 0.0 | 0 | 0.16 | 0.0 |
| OTHER FEMALE GENITAL | 0 | 0.04 | 0.0 | 0 | 0.0 | 0.0 | 0 | 0.04 | 0.0 |
| PROSTATE | 3 | 1.30 | 2.30 | 3 | 1.30 | 2.30 | 0 | 0.0 | 0.0 |
| TESTIS | 0 | 0.02 | 0.0 | 0 | 0.02 | 0.0 | 0 | 0.0 | 0.0 |
| OTHER MALE GENITAL | 0 | 0.03 | 0.0 | 0 | 0.03 | 0.0 | 0 | 0.0 | 0.0 |
| KIDNEY AND URETER | 1 | 0.22 | 4.50 | 0 | 0.17 | 0.0 | 1 | 0.05 | 18.32 |
| BLADDER | 0 | 0.65 | 0.0 | 0 | 0.53 | 0.0 | 0 | 0.11 | 0.0 |
| MELANOMA OF SKIN | 0 | 0.07 | 0.0 | 0 | 0.04 | 0.0 | 0 | 0.03 | 0.0 |
| EYE | 0 | 0.02 | 0.0 | 0 | 0.01 | 0.0 | 0 | 0.01 | 0.0 |
| NERVOUS SYSTEM | 0 | 0.10 | 0.0 | 0 | 0.07 | 0.0 | 0 | 0.03 | 0.0 |
| THYROID | 0 | 0.05 | 0.0 | 0 | 0.02 | 0.0 | 0 | 0.03 | 0.0 |
| BONE | 0 | 0.03 | 0.0 | 0 | 0.02 | 0.0 | 0 | 0.01 | 0.0 |
| SOFT TISSUE | 0 | 0.07 | 0.0 | 0 | 0.05 | 0.0 | 0 | 0.02 | 0.0 |
| LYMPHOMAS & MYELOMA | 1 | 0.30 | 3.38 | 1 | 0.20 | 4.92 | 0 | 0.09 | 0.0 |
| LEUKEMIAS | 0 | 0.31 | 0.0 | 0 | 0.22 | 0.0 | 0 | 0.09 | 0.0 |
| OTHER SITES | 0 | 0.62 | 0.0 | 0 | 0.40 | 0.0 | 0 | 0.21 | 0.0 |
| TOTAL | 13 | 11.35 | 1.15 | 7 | 7.68 | 0.91 | 6 | 3.67 | 1.64 |

Table 50. Subsequent primary sites with excesses

FIRST PRIMARY SITE - NOSE,NASAL CAVITIES,MIDDLE EAR,AND ACCESSORY SINUSES

| | TOTAL | | | YEARS < 1 | | | YEARS 1-5 | | | YEARS > 5 | | |
|---|---|---|---|---|---|---|---|---|---|---|---|---|
| | NUMBER OF PERSONS= 338 PERSON-YRS OF OBSERVATION= 1207.2 | | | NUMBER OF PERSONS= 338 PERSON-YRS OF OBSERVATION= 266.8 | | | NUMBER OF PERSONS= 201 PERSON-YRS OF OBSERVATION= 465.2 | | | NUMBER OF PERSONS= 78 PERSCN-YRS OF OBSERVATION= 475.2 | | |
| SUBSEQUENT PRIMARY SITES | OBS | EXP | OBS/EXP | OBS | EXP | OBS/EXP | OBS | EXP | OBS/EXP | OES | EXP | OBS/EXP |
| BREAST | 4 | 0.87 | 4.60* | 0 | 0.18 | 0.0 | 2 | 0.35 | 5.76 | 2 | 0.35 | 5.79 |
| PROSTATE | 3 | 1.30 | 2.30 | 0 | 0.28 | 0.0 | 3 | 0.45 | 6.70* | C | 0.58 | 0.0 |

Table 51. Histologic confirmation of multiple primary malignancies

FIRST PRIMARY SITE - NOSE, NASAL CAVITIES, MIDDLE EAR, AND ACCESSORY SINUSES

| Subsequent primary site | Both tumors microscopically confirmed | | Only 1st tumor microscopically confirmed | | Only 2nd tumor microscopically confirmed | | Neither tumor microscopically confirmed | |
|---|---|---|---|---|---|---|---|---|
| | No. | % | No. | % | No. | % | No. | % |
| BREAST | 3 | 75.0 | 1 | 25.0 | 0 | 0.0 | 0 | 0.0 |
| PROSTATE | 0 | 0.0 | 2 | 66.7 | 0 | 0.0 | 1 | 33.3 |

Table 52. Subsequent multiple primary malignancies in patients with an index malignant tumor of the larynx

FIRST PRIMARY SITE - LARYNX

| SUBSEQUENT PRIMARY SITES | TOTAL | | | MALES | | | FEMALES | | |
|---|---|---|---|---|---|---|---|---|---|
| | NUMBER OF PERSONS= 1731 PERSON-YRS OF OBSERVATION = 6745.0 | | | NUMBER OF PERSONS= 1587 PERSON-YRS OF OBSERVATION = 6195.7 | | | NUMBER OF PERSONS= 144 PERSON-YRS OF OBSERVATION = 549.2 | | |
| | OBS | EXP | OBS/EXP | OBS | EXP | OBS/EXP | OBS | EXP | OBS/EXP |
| LIP | 0 | 1.10 | 0.0 | 0 | 1.10 | 0.0 | 0 | 0.00 | 0.0 |
| TONGUE | 7 | 0.96 | 7.29** | 7 | 0.95 | 7.37** | 0 | 0.01 | 0.0 |
| SALIVARY GLAND | 0 | 0.22 | 0.0 | 0 | 0.21 | 0.0 | 0 | 0.01 | 0.0 |
| MOUTH | 4 | 1.17 | 3.41 | 4 | 1.16 | 3.46 | 0 | 0.02 | 0.0 |
| PHARYNX | 4 | 1.22 | 3.29 | 4 | 1.20 | 3.33 | 0 | 0.02 | 0.0 |
| ESOPHAGUS | 3 | 2.16 | 1.39 | 3 | 2.14 | 1.40 | 0 | 0.02 | 0.0 |
| STOMACH | 8 | 7.09 | 1.13 | 8 | 6.86 | 1.17 | 0 | 0.23 | 0.0 |
| SMALL INTESTINE | 2 | 0.27 | 7.45 | 1 | 0.25 | 3.93 | 1 | 0.01 | 70.12* |
| COLON | 14 | 8.87 | 1.58 | 12 | 8.31 | 1.44 | 2 | 0.56 | 3.58 |
| RECTUM | 9 | 5.61 | 1.60 | 9 | 5.38 | 1.67 | 0 | 0.24 | 0.0 |
| LIVER & BILIARY PASS | 3 | 1.63 | 1.84 | 3 | 1.52 | 1.97 | 0 | 0.11 | 0.0 |
| PANCREAS | 6 | 2.89 | 2.08 | 6 | 2.77 | 2.17 | 0 | 0.12 | 0.0 |
| NOSE AND SINUSES | 1 | 0.17 | 5.98 | 1 | 0.16 | 6.23 | 0 | 0.01 | 0.0 |
| LARYNX | 1 | 1.81 | 0.55 | 1 | 1.80 | 0.56 | 0 | 0.01 | 0.0 |
| LUNG AND BRONCHUS | 27 | 10.55 | 2.56** | 26 | 10.45 | 2.49** | 1 | 0.10 | 9.66 |
| OTHER RESP | 0 | 0.15 | 0.0 | 0 | 0.15 | 0.0 | 0 | 0.00 | 0.0 |
| BREAST | 2 | 1.18 | 1.70 | 1 | 0.19 | 5.26 | 1 | 0.99 | 1.01 |
| CERVIX UTERI | 1 | 0.27 | 3.69 | 0 | 0.0 | 0.0 | 1 | 0.27 | 3.69 |
| CORPUS UTERI | 0 | 0.22 | 0.0 | 0 | 0.0 | 0.0 | 0 | 0.22 | 0.0 |
| UTERUS,UNSPEC | 0 | 0.10 | 0.0 | 0 | 0.0 | 0.0 | 0 | 0.10 | 0.0 |
| OVARY | 0 | 0.20 | 0.0 | 0 | 0.0 | 0.0 | 0 | 0.20 | 0.0 |
| OTHER FEMALE GENITAL | 0 | 0.04 | 0.0 | 0 | 0.0 | 0.0 | 0 | 0.04 | 0.0 |
| PROSTATE | 27 | 12.30 | 2.20** | 27 | 12.30 | 2.20** | 0 | 0.0 | 0.0 |
| TESTIS | 0 | 0.14 | 0.0 | 0 | 0.14 | 0.0 | 0 | 0.0 | 0.0 |
| OTHER MALE GENITAL | 0 | 0.26 | 0.0 | 0 | 0.26 | 0.0 | 0 | 0.0 | 0.0 |
| KIDNEY AND URETER | 1 | 1.75 | 0.57 | 1 | 1.69 | 0.59 | 0 | 0.06 | 0.0 |
| BLADDER | 9 | 5.42 | 1.66 | 9 | 5.31 | 1.69 | 0 | 0.11 | 0.0 |
| MELANOMA OF SKIN | 1 | 0.43 | 2.31 | 1 | 0.40 | 2.50 | 0 | 0.03 | 0.0 |
| EYE | 0 | 0.14 | 0.0 | 0 | 0.13 | 0.0 | 0 | 0.01 | 0.0 |
| NERVOUS SYSTEM | 0 | 0.68 | 0.0 | 0 | 0.64 | 0.0 | 0 | 0.04 | 0.0 |
| THYROID | 0 | 0.24 | 0.0 | 0 | 0.21 | 0.0 | 0 | 0.03 | 0.0 |
| BONE | 0 | 0.18 | 0.0 | 0 | 0.17 | 0.0 | 0 | 0.01 | 0.0 |
| SOFT TISSUE | 0 | 0.52 | 0.0 | 0 | 0.49 | 0.0 | 0 | 0.03 | 0.0 |
| LYMPHOMAS & MYELOMA | 4 | 2.07 | 1.93 | 4 | 1.96 | 2.04 | 0 | 0.11 | 0.0 |
| LEUKEMIAS | 3 | 2.30 | 1.31 | 3 | 2.20 | 1.36 | 0 | 0.09 | 0.0 |
| OTHER SITES | 3 | 4.22 | 0.71 | 3 | 4.00 | 0.75 | 0 | 0.22 | 0.0 |
| TOTAL | 140 | 78.54 | 1.78** | 134 | 74.51 | 1.80** | 6 | 4.03 | 1.49 |

Table 53. Subsequent primary sites with excesses

FIRST PRIMARY SITE - LARYNX

| SUBSEQUENT PRIMARY SITES | TOTAL | | | YEARS < 1 | | | YEARS 1-5 | | | YEARS > 5 | | |
|---|---|---|---|---|---|---|---|---|---|---|---|---|
| | NUMBER OF PERSONS= 1731 PERSON-YRS OF OBSERVATION= 6745.0 | | | NUMBER OF PERSONS= 1731 PERSON-YRS OF OBSERVATION= 1437.2 | | | NUMBER OF PERSONS= 1174 PERSON-YRS OF OBSERVATION= 2916.1 | | | NUMBER OF PERSONS= 476 PERSON-YRS OF OBSERVATION= 2391.7 | | |
| | OBS | EXP | OBS/EXP | OBS | EXP | OBS/EXP | OBS | EXP | OBS/EXP | OBS | EXP | OBS/EXP |
| TONGUE | 7 | 0.96 | 7.29** | 2 | 0.19 | 10.77* | 3 | 0.39 | 7.61* | 2 | 0.38 | 5.26 |
| PHARYNX | 4 | 1.22 | 3.29 | 2 | 0.23 | 8.64* | 1 | 0.50 | 1.99 | 1 | 0.48 | 2.08 |
| SMALL INTESTINE | 2 | 0.27 | 7.45 | 2 | 0.05 | 39.93** | 0 | 0.11 | 0.0 | 0 | 0.11 | 0.0 |
| LUNG AND BRONCHUS | 27 | 10.55 | 2.56** | 2 | 1.91 | 1.05 | 14 | 4.32 | 3.24** | 11 | 4.33 | 2.54* |
| PROSTATE | 27 | 12.30 | 2.20** | 7 | 2.05 | 3.41* | 9 | 4.64 | 1.94 | 11 | 5.61 | 1.96 |
| BLADDER | 9 | 5.42 | 1.66 | 0 | 0.96 | 0.0 | 7 | 2.15 | 3.26* | 2 | 2.31 | 0.86 |

Table 54. Histologic confirmation of multiple primary malignancies

FIRST PRIMARY SITE - LARYNX

| Subsequent primary site | Both tumor microscopically confirmed | | Only 1st tumor microscopically confirmed | | Only 2nd tumor microscopically confirmed | | Neither tumor microscopically confirmed | |
|---|---|---|---|---|---|---|---|---|
| | No. | % | No. | % | No. | % | No. | % |
| TONGUE | 5 | 71.4 | 1 | 14.3 | 1 | 14.3 | 0 | 0.0 |
| PHARYNX | 4 | 100.0 | 0 | 0.0 | 0 | 0.0 | 0 | 0.0 |
| SMALL INTESTINE | 2 | 100.0 | 0 | 0.0 | 0 | 0.0 | 0 | 0.0 |
| LUNG AND BRONCHUS | 22 | 81.5 | 3 | 11.1 | 1 | 3.7 | 1 | 3.7 |
| PROSTATE | 25 | 92.6 | 2 | 7.4 | 0 | 0.0 | 0 | 0.0 |
| BLADDER | 8 | 88.9 | 1 | 11.1 | 0 | 0.0 | 0 | 0.0 |

Table 55. Subsequent multiple malignancies in patients with an index malignant tumor of the lungs and bronchus

FIRST PRIMARY SITE - LUNG AND BRONCHUS

| | TOTAL | | | MALES | | | FEMALES | | |
|---|---|---|---|---|---|---|---|---|---|
| | NUMBER OF PERSONS= 7983 PERSON-YRS OF OBSERVATION = 7142.7 | | | NUMBER OF PERSONS= 6783 PERSON-YRS OF OBSERVATION = 5940.2 | | | NUMBER OF PERSONS= 1200 PERSON-YRS OF OBSERVATION = 1202.5 | | |
| SUBSEQUENT PRIMARY SITES | OBS | EXP | OBS/EXP | OBS | EXP | OBS/EXP | OBS | EXP | OBS/EXP |
| LIP | 1 | 0.92 | 1.09 | 1 | 0.91 | 1.10 | 0 | 0.01 | 0.0 |
| TONGUE | 2 | 0.85 | 2.37 | 2 | 0.82 | 2.43 | 0 | 0.02 | 0.0 |
| SALIVARY GLAND | 0 | 0.21 | 0.0 | 0 | 0.18 | 0.0 | 0 | 0.02 | 0.0 |
| MOUTH | 1 | 1.03 | 0.97 | 1 | 0.99 | 1.01 | 0 | 0.04 | 0.0 |
| PHARYNX | 4 | 1.13 | 3.54 | 3 | 1.09 | 2.74 | 1 | 0.03 | 29.50 |
| ESOPHAGUS | 1 | 1.91 | 0.52 | 1 | 1.87 | 0.54 | 0 | 0.05 | 0.0 |
| STOMACH | 2 | 5.91 | 0.34 | 2 | 5.41 | 0.37 | 0 | 0.51 | 0.0 |
| SMALL INTESTINE | 0 | 0.26 | 0.0 | 0 | 0.23 | 0.0 | 0 | 0.03 | 0.0 |
| COLON | 11 | 8.13 | 1.35 | 11 | 6.90 | 1.59 | 0 | 1.23 | 0.0 |
| RECTUM | 4 | 4.99 | 0.80 | 3 | 4.46 | 0.67 | 1 | 0.52 | 1.91 |
| LIVER & BILIARY PASS | 2 | 1.52 | 1.31 | 2 | 1.28 | 1.56 | 0 | 0.24 | 0.0 |
| PANCREAS | 6 | 2.61 | 2.30 | 6 | 2.35 | 2.55 | 0 | 0.27 | 0.0 |
| NOSE AND SINUSES | 0 | 0.14 | 0.0 | 0 | 0.13 | 0.0 | 0 | 0.01 | 0.0 |
| LARYNX | 4 | 1.70 | 2.36 | 4 | 1.68 | 2.38 | 0 | 0.02 | 0.0 |
| LUNG AND BRONCHUS | 10 | 10.52 | 0.95 | 9 | 10.29 | 0.87 | 1 | 0.23 | 4.32 |
| OTHER RESP | 0 | 0.15 | 0.0 | 0 | 0.15 | 0.0 | 0 | 0.01 | 0.0 |
| BREAST | 2 | 2.30 | 0.87 | 0 | 0.17 | 0.0 | 2 | 2.13 | 0.94 |
| CERVIX UTERI | 1 | 0.57 | 1.75 | 0 | 0.0 | 0.0 | 1 | 0.57 | 1.75 |
| CORPUS UTERI | 1 | 0.48 | 2.09 | 0 | 0.0 | 0.0 | 1 | 0.48 | 2.09 |
| UTERUS,UNSPEC | 0 | 0.21 | 0.0 | 0 | 0.0 | 0.0 | 0 | 0.21 | 0.0 |
| OVARY | 2 | 0.43 | 4.64 | 0 | 0.0 | 0.0 | 2 | 0.43 | 4.64 |
| OTHER FEMALE GENITAL | 0 | 0.09 | 0.0 | 0 | 0.0 | 0.0 | 0 | 0.09 | 0.0 |
| PROSTATE | 32 | 9.31 | 3.44** | 32 | 9.31 | 3.44** | 0 | 0.0 | 0.0 |
| TESTIS | 0 | 0.13 | 0.0 | 0 | 0.13 | 0.0 | 0 | 0.0 | 0.0 |
| OTHER MALE GENITAL | 0 | 0.22 | 0.0 | 0 | 0.22 | 0.0 | 0 | 0.0 | 0.0 |
| KIDNEY AND URETER | 10 | 1.66 | 6.02** | 10 | 1.53 | 6.53** | 0 | 0.13 | 0.0 |
| BLADDER | 6 | 4.80 | 1.25 | 6 | 4.56 | 1.32 | 0 | 0.24 | 0.0 |
| MELANOMA OF SKIN | 1 | 0.44 | 2.28 | 1 | 0.37 | 2.74 | 0 | 0.07 | 0.0 |
| EYE | 0 | 0.13 | 0.0 | 0 | 0.11 | 0.0 | 0 | 0.02 | 0.0 |
| NERVOUS SYSTEM | 0 | 0.74 | 0.0 | 0 | 0.65 | 0.0 | 0 | 0.09 | 0.0 |
| THYROID | 1 | 0.26 | 3.89 | 1 | 0.19 | 5.29 | 0 | 0.07 | 0.0 |
| BONE | 0 | 0.17 | 0.0 | 0 | 0.14 | 0.0 | 0 | 0.02 | 0.0 |
| SOFT TISSUE | 1 | 0.51 | 1.94 | 1 | 0.45 | 2.21 | 0 | 0.06 | 0.0 |
| LYMPHOMAS & MYELOMA | 2 | 2.04 | 0.98 | 1 | 1.80 | 0.56 | 1 | 0.24 | 4.10 |
| LEUKEMIAS | 3 | 2.11 | 1.42 | 3 | 1.90 | 1.58 | 0 | 0.21 | 0.0 |
| OTHER SITES | 2 | 4.07 | 0.49 | 1 | 3.57 | 0.28 | 1 | 0.49 | 2.03 |
| TOTAL | 112 | 72.67 | 1.54** | 101 | 63.86 | 1.58** | 11 | 8.81 | 1.25 |

Table 56. Subsequent primary sites with excesses

FIRST PRIMARY SITE - LUNG AND BRONCHUS

| SUBSEQUENT PRIMARY SITES | TOTAL<br>NUMBER OF PERSONS= 7983<br>PERSON-YRS OF OBSERVATION= 7142.7 | | | YEARS < 1<br>NUMBER OF PERSONS= 7983<br>PERSON-YRS OF OBSERVATION= 3833.0 | | | YEARS 1-5<br>NUMBER OF PERSONS= 1782<br>PERSON-YRS OF OBSERVATION= 2481.4 | | | YEARS > 5<br>NUMBER OF PERSONS= 248<br>PERSON-YRS OF OBSERVATION= 828.3 | | |
|---|---|---|---|---|---|---|---|---|---|---|---|---|
| | OBS | EXP | OBS/EXP | OBS | EXP | OBS/EXP | OBS | EXP | OBS/EXP | OBS | EXP | OBS/EXP |
| LARYNX | 4 | 1.70 | 2.36 | 0 | 0.88 | 0.0 | 2 | 0.61 | 3.30 | 2 | 0.22 | 9.27* |
| OVARY | 2 | 0.43 | 4.64 | 0 | 0.21 | 0.0 | 2 | 0.15 | 13.17* | 0 | 0.07 | 0.0 |
| PROSTATE | 32 | 9.31 | 3.44** | 21 | 4.80 | 4.37** | 8 | 3.25 | 2.46* | 3 | 1.26 | 2.39 |
| KIDNEY AND URETER | 10 | 1.66 | 6.02** | 4 | 0.86 | 4.67* | 5 | 0.59 | 8.49** | 1 | 0.21 | 4.65 |

Table 57. Histologic confirmation of multiple primary malignancies

FIRST PRIMARY SITE - LUNG AND BRONCHUS

| Subsequent primary site | Both tumors microscopically confirmed | | Only 1st tumor microscopically confirmed | | Only 2nd tumor microscopically confirmed | | Neither tumor microscopically confirmed | |
|---|---|---|---|---|---|---|---|---|
| | No. | % | No. | % | No. | % | No. | % |
| LARYNX | 4 | 100.0 | 0 | 0.0 | 0 | 0.0 | 0 | 0.0 |
| OVARY | 2 | 100.0 | 0 | 0.0 | 0 | 0.0 | 0 | 0.0 |
| PROSTATE | 28 | 87.5 | 2 | 6.3 | 0 | 0.0 | 2 | 6.3 |
| KIDNEY AND URETER | 8 | 80.0 | 2 | 20.0 | 0 | 0.0 | 0 | 0.0 |

Table 58. Subsequent multiple primary malignancies in patients with an index malignant tumor of other respiratory organs

FIRST PRIMARY SITE - MEDIASTINUM AND RESPIRATORY SYSTEM UNSPECIFIED

| SUBSEQUENT PRIMARY SITES | TOTAL | | | MALES | | | FEMALES | | |
|---|---|---|---|---|---|---|---|---|---|
| | NUMBER OF PERSONS= 218 PERSON-YRS OF OBSERVATION = 342.0 | | | NUMBER OF PERSONS= 149 PERSON-YRS OF OBSERVATION = 257.2 | | | NUMBER OF PERSONS= 69 PERSON-YRS OF OBSERVATION = 84.8 | | |
| | OBS | EXP | OBS/EXP | OBS | EXP | OBS/EXP | OBS | EXP | OBS/EXP |
| LIP | 0 | 0.01 | 0.0 | 0 | 0.01 | 0.0 | 0 | 0.00 | 0.0 |
| TONGUE | 0 | 0.02 | 0.0 | 0 | 0.01 | 0.0 | 0 | 0.00 | 0.0 |
| SALIVARY GLAND | 0 | 0.00 | 0.0 | 0 | 0.00 | 0.0 | 0 | 0.00 | 0.0 |
| MOUTH | 0 | 0.02 | 0.0 | 0 | 0.02 | 0.0 | 0 | 0.00 | 0.0 |
| PHARYNX | 0 | 0.02 | 0.0 | 0 | 0.02 | 0.0 | 0 | 0.00 | 0.0 |
| ESOPHAGUS | 0 | 0.03 | 0.0 | 0 | 0.03 | 0.0 | 0 | 0.00 | 0.0 |
| STOMACH | 1 | 0.09 | 10.72 | 1 | 0.08 | 12.57 | 0 | 0.01 | 0.0 |
| SMALL INTESTINE | 0 | 0.00 | 0.0 | 0 | 0.00 | 0.0 | 0 | 0.00 | 0.0 |
| COLON | 1 | 0.13 | 7.90 | 1 | 0.09 | 10.54 | 0 | 0.03 | 0.0 |
| RECTUM | 0 | 0.08 | 0.0 | 0 | 0.07 | 0.0 | 0 | 0.02 | 0.0 |
| LIVER & BILIARY PASS | 0 | 0.02 | 0.0 | 0 | 0.02 | 0.0 | 0 | 0.01 | 0.0 |
| PANCREAS | 0 | 0.04 | 0.0 | 0 | 0.03 | 0.0 | 0 | 0.01 | 0.0 |
| NOSE AND SINUSES | 0 | 0.00 | 0.0 | 0 | 0.00 | 0.0 | 0 | 0.00 | 0.0 |
| LARYNX | 0 | 0.03 | 0.0 | 0 | 0.03 | 0.0 | 0 | 0.00 | 0.0 |
| LUNG AND BRONCHUS | 1 | 0.16 | 6.29 | 1 | 0.15 | 6.60 | 0 | 0.01 | 0.0 |
| OTHER RESP | 0 | 0.00 | 0.0 | 0 | 0.00 | 0.0 | 0 | 0.00 | 0.0 |
| BREAST | 1 | 0.09 | 10.68 | 0 | 0.00 | 0.0 | 1 | 0.09 | 11.01 |
| CERVIX UTERI | 0 | 0.04 | 0.0 | 0 | 0.0 | 0.0 | 0 | 0.04 | 0.0 |
| CORPUS UTERI | 0 | 0.02 | 0.0 | 0 | 0.0 | 0.0 | 0 | 0.02 | 0.0 |
| UTERUS,UNSPEC | 0 | 0.01 | 0.0 | 0 | 0.0 | 0.0 | 0 | 0.01 | 0.0 |
| OVARY | 0 | 0.02 | 0.0 | 0 | 0.0 | 0.0 | 0 | 0.02 | 0.0 |
| OTHER FEMALE GENITAL | 0 | 0.00 | 0.0 | 0 | 0.0 | 0.0 | 0 | 0.00 | 0.0 |
| PROSTATE | 1 | 0.10 | 10.19 | 1 | 0.10 | 10.19 | 0 | 0.0 | 0.0 |
| TESTIS | 0 | 0.01 | 0.0 | 0 | 0.01 | 0.0 | 0 | 0.0 | 0.0 |
| OTHER MALE GENITAL | 0 | 0.00 | 0.0 | 0 | 0.00 | 0.0 | 0 | 0.0 | 0.0 |
| KIDNEY AND URETER | 0 | 0.03 | 0.0 | 0 | 0.02 | 0.0 | 0 | 0.00 | 0.0 |
| BLADDER | 0 | 0.07 | 0.0 | 0 | 0.06 | 0.0 | 0 | 0.01 | 0.0 |
| MELANOMA OF SKIN | 0 | 0.01 | 0.0 | 0 | 0.01 | 0.0 | 0 | 0.00 | 0.0 |
| EYE | 0 | 0.00 | 0.0 | 0 | 0.00 | 0.0 | 0 | 0.00 | 0.0 |
| NERVOUS SYSTEM | 0 | 0.02 | 0.0 | 0 | 0.02 | 0.0 | 0 | 0.01 | 0.0 |
| THYROID | 0 | 0.01 | 0.0 | 0 | 0.00 | 0.0 | 0 | 0.00 | 0.0 |
| BONE | 1 | 0.00 | 223.45** | 0 | 0.00 | 0.0 | 1 | 0.00 | 1229.51** |
| SOFT TISSUE | 0 | 0.01 | 0.0 | 0 | 0.01 | 0.0 | 0 | 0.00 | 0.0 |
| LYMPHOMAS & MYELOMA | 0 | 0.04 | 0.0 | 0 | 0.03 | 0.0 | 0 | 0.01 | 0.0 |
| LEUKEMIAS | 0 | 0.04 | 0.0 | 0 | 0.03 | 0.0 | 0 | 0.01 | 0.0 |
| OTHER SITES | 0 | 0.07 | 0.0 | 0 | 0.05 | 0.0 | 0 | 0.01 | 0.0 |
| TOTAL | 6 | 1.25 | 4.81** | 4 | 0.93 | 4.31* | 2 | 0.32 | 6.28 |

Table 59. Subsequent primary sites with excesses

FIRST PRIMARY SITE - MEDIASTINUM AND RESPIRATORY SYSTEM UNSPECIFIED

| | TOTAL | | | YEARS < 1 | | | YEARS 1-5 | | | YEARS > 5 | | |
|---|---|---|---|---|---|---|---|---|---|---|---|---|
| | NUMBER OF PERSONS= 218<br>PERSON-YRS OF OBSERVATION= 342.0 | | | NUMBER OF PERSONS= 218<br>PERSON-YRS OF OBSERVATION= 118.7 | | | NUMBER OF PERSONS= 65<br>PERSON-YRS OF OBSERVATION= 134.4 | | | NUMBER OF PERSONS= 18<br>PERSON-YRS OF OBSERVATION= 88.8 | | |
| SUBSEQUENT PRIMARY SITES | OBS | EXP | OBS/EXP | OBS | EXP | OBS/EXP | OBS | EXP | OBS/EXP | OBS | EXP | OBS/EXP |
| COLON | 1 | 0.13 | 7.90 | 0 | 0.06 | 0.0 | 0 | 0.05 | 0.0 | 1 | 0.02 | 57.68* |
| BONE | 1 | 0.00 | 223.45** | 0 | 0.00 | 0.0 | 1 | 0.00 | 650.02** | 0 | 0.00 | 0.0 |

Table 60. Histologic confirmation of multiple primary malignancies

FIRST PRIMARY SITE - MEDIASTINUM AND RESPIRATORY SYSTEM UNSPECIFIED

| Subsequent primary site | Both tumors microscopically confirmed | | Only 1st tumor microscopically confirmed | | Only 2nd tumor microscopically confirmed | | Neither tumor microscopically confirmed | |
|---|---|---|---|---|---|---|---|---|
| | No. | % | No. | % | No. | % | No. | % |
| COLON | 0 | 0.0 | 0 | 0.0 | 1 | 100.0 | 0 | 0.0 |
| BONE | 1 | 100.0 | 0 | 0.0 | 0 | 0.0 | 0 | 0.0 |

Table 61. Summary of site-group pairs with an excess of observed-over-expected subsequent primary malignancies: index tumors of the respiratory system

I. Possibly artifact

- Nose/sinuses ------------------------> Prostate
- Larynx ------------------------------> Prostate
- Lung/bronchus -----------------------> Prostate
- Nose/sinuses ------------------------> Breast
- Larynx ------------------------------> Small intestine
- Lung/bronchus -----------------------> Ovary
- Other respiratory organs ------------> Colon
- Other respiratory organs ------------> Bone

II. Possibly real

A. In organs within the same system

- Larynx <-----------------------------> Lung/bronchus

B. In organs related structurally or functionally

- Larynx ------------------------------> Tongue
- Larynx ------------------------------> Pharynx

C. In organs apparently unrelated structurally or functionally

- Larynx ------------------------------> Bladder
- Lung/bronchus -----------------------> Kidney/ureter

Table 62. Common metastatic sites for primary malignant tumors of the respiratory system (HOLLAND and FREI, 1973; WILLIS, 1973; RUBIN, 1974)

| Anatomic location of the primary malignant tumor | Common metastatic sites |
|---|---|
| Paranasal sinuses | Cervical nodes; orbit of eye |
| Glottis | Cervical nodes |
| Larynx | Jugulo-digastric nodes, vocal cord |
| Lung/bronchus | Ipsilateral hilar, contralateral hilar, mediastinal, scalene, and cervical lymph nodes; opposite lung; brain; bone (skeleton); adrenals; eye; thyroid; liver |

# Chapter 9

# Index Tumors of the Breast and Reproductive Organs

Population Studied. 130 males and 18,010 females with breast cancer and 8,228 males and 17,405 females with cancer of the genital organs were followed for the subsequent development of independent primary malignant neoplasms; 2,259 such subsequent neoplasms were diagnosed. The cohort of patients with cancer of the breast or genital organs contributed 218,038 person-years of observation.

Results. Detailed tabulations by site are presented in Tables 63-91. The reader is referred to Chapter 5 for a general explanation of the items in these tables.

Summary of Findings. Site-group pairs with a statistically significant excess of observed-over-expected subsequent primary cancers are categorized in Table 92 on the basis of possible relationships between the anatomic sites containing these cancers. In addition, possible artifactual relationships, based on relatively few cases and/or with no confirmation from other reports, are emphasized. In most instances, index cancers of the male genital organs are considered after index malignancies of the female genital organs. Table 93 outlines site-group pairs with a statistically significant deficiency of observed-over-expected subsequent primary cancers.

Discussion. Table 94 presents the common metastatic sites for cancers arising within the breast and genital organs. These data, used in conjunction with the site-specific tabulations of the percentage of multiple primary malignancies with histologic confirmation, are useful in distinguishing real from artifactual associations.

The relationships outlined in category I of Table 92 are thought to be spurious. The excess risk of tongue cancer in breast cancer patients is based on only five observed cases; in only three of the five patients are both neoplasms histologically confirmed. The association between breast and bladder cancer, although based on 25 observed cases, is statistically significant in only one time interval, namely, 1-5 years following the breast cancer diagnosis. Without documentation from other published reports it is felt that the statistical significance of this relationship represents a chance occurrence.

The excess risk of cancer of other/unspecified sites in patients with a malignancy of the uterine cervix is significant in only one time interval, and has not been observed in other studies of cancer of the uterine cervix. Also, 17% of the extra-uterine malignancies were not histologically verified. The remaining site-group pairs in category I are based on fewer than five observed cases and are unconfirmed by other reports.

The excess risk of subsequent breast cancer in breast cancer patients is well described (ROBBINS and BERG, 1964; NEWELL et al., 1974c).

Excesses of observed-over-expected second primary cancers in the same or paired organs or occurring within the same organ system might be explained on the basis of related tissue being exposed to the same oncogenic factors (genetic and/or environmental). These are shown in category IIA. There are several case reports in the literature documenting the rather common occurrence of this phenomenon within the female genital organs (WOODRUFF and JULIAN, 1969; JIMERSON and MERRILL, 1970; BLOOMFIELD and SAMIMY, 1972; RAJHAVJN and KURJAK, 1973; NEWELL et al., 1974c). One group of authors has suggested that excessive hormone production by an ovarian neoplasm may induce an endometrial malignancy (BENISCH and TOKER, 1973).

A common carcinogenic agent acting on related tissue could explain the increased risk of malignancies of other/unspecified male genital organs in patients with prostatic cancer. Although the chance of mistaking metastatic disease for an independent neoplasm is great in closely related organs, all five patients exhibiting cancers of both the prostate and other/unspecified male genital organs had both malignancies confirmed microscopically.

Category IIB includes site-group pairs which are functionally related. The associations of these site-group pairs are supported by other investigations (BAILAR, 1963; MACMAHON and AUSTIN, 1969; VONGTAMA et al., 1970; SCHOTTENFELD and BERG, 1971; SILVERMAN et al., 1972; NEWELL et al., 1975). To explain the relationship between cancer of the breast and either primary cancer of the corpus uteri or the ovary, the role of possible hormone influences should be considered. It has been shown that castration of mice of high breast cancer strains results in a reduced incidence of this malignancy in these mice (CORI, 1927). Other investigators have shown that menopause occurs later in women who had breast cancer than in control populations (OLCH, 1937; HEIBERG and HEIBERG, 1940). Some studies give anatomic evidence of high estrogen levels associated more often with endometrial or breast carcinoma patients than with normal controls (MORRIS and SCULLY, 1958; MARCUSE, 1966).

The group at high risk for one cancer may also be at high risk for the other cancer for demographic factors other than age and sex, which were considered in the computation of expected numbers of subsequent primary cancers. Numerous other studies have shown that patients with breast cancer are more frequently unmarried, or if married, have lower pregnancy rates than comparable controls (HEIBERG and HEIBERG, 1940; HARNETT, 1948; GILLIAM, 1951; WYNDER et al., 1960; LILIENFELD, 1963). Similarly, endometrial cancer patients have a high incidence of infertility (SPEERT, 1949; SOMMERS et al., 1949; DOCKERTY et al., 1955; CORSCADEN, 1962).

In organs apparently unrelated functionally or anatomically, the following site-group pairs revealed a two-way association:

uterine corpus and colon
ovary and colon

These findings are in agreement with the results of several investigations (BAILAR, 1963; SCHOTTENFELD et al., 1969; SCHOTTENFELD and BERG, 1971). In only one of these previously published series, based on the experience of the Memorial Hospital for Cancer and Allied Diseases, were the numbers large enough to reach statistical significance (SCHOTTENFELD and BERG, 1971). The possibility of selection bias in terms of the patient population served by Memorial Hospital must be considered.

The present findings from a statewide, population-based registry add support to the possible etiologic significance in females of the association among cancers of the colon, uterine corpus, and ovary. The association between cancer of the uterine corpus and colon has been reported in a number of studies of intrafamilial cancer (HAUSER and WELLER, 1936; SAVAGE, 1956; LYNCH et al., 1967).

Age-adjusted incidence data for various ethnic groups within the Israeli population revealed a correlation between cancer of the colon and ovary (STEINITZ, 1967). Several investigations suggesting a higher incidence of infertility among women with colon cancer and among women with endometrial cancer have been described in Chapter 7 (SPEERT, 1949; SOMMERS et al., 1949; DOCKERTY et al., 1955; CORSCADEN, 1962; ACHESON et al., submitted for publication). Also, international mortality data for cancer of the colon and uterine corpus are closely correlated (DUNHAM and BAILAR, 1968).

The excess risk of colon cancer among breast cancer patients in Connecticut is limited to the time period greater than 5 years after the breast cancer diagnosis. A review of the experience of Memorial Hospital in New York revealed an excess risk of breast cancer among women with colon cancer, but because of small numbers this was not statistically significant (SCHOTTENFELD et al., 1969). With regard to explaining this association, several reports have shown that patients with breast cancer are more frequently unmarried, or if married, have lower pregnancy rates than comparable controls (HEIBERG and HEIBERG, 1940; HARNETT, 1948; GILLIAM, 1951; WYNDER et al., 1960; LILIENFELD, 1963). Thus infertility or reduced fertility is associated with an increased risk of cancer of the female breast, colon, ovary, and uterine corpus. WYNDER hypothesized that dietary habits have a direct effect on colon cancer risk and an indirect effect (mediated through hormonal mechanisms) on breast cancer risk (WYNDER et al., 1967).

The excess risk of soft-tissue malignancies in breast cancer patients is concentrated in the time interval beginning 5 years after the diagnosis of the breast cancer. These soft-tissue neoplasms are primarily lymphangiosarcomas of the upper extremity, a known sequela of radical mastectomy and resulting lymphedema. This entity was first described in 1948 (STEWART and TREVES, 1948).

For cases in which an association is unidirectional, as exemplified by the relationship between breast cancer and soft-tissue malignancies, it may be that something unique about patients with one cancer predisposes them to develop another cancer. One such unique factor may be treatment (i.e., treatment for the first cancer inducing the later cancer). The carcinogenic effects of radiation, often used in the treatment of genital cancer, should be considered as a possible cause of the later primary cancer (NOVAK and WOODRUFF, 1959; WILLSON et al., 1963). That irradiation for cancer of the uterine corpus or cervix may induce a cancer in a nearby structure, such as the rectum, is therefore not inconceivable (SLAUGHTER and SOUTHWICK, 1957; SMITH, 1962; MACMAHON and ROWE, 1971). In order to explore these hypotheses more fully, the excess risk of rectal cancer following a uterine malignancy (both uterine cervix and uterine corpus) was analyzed by time interval between the first and later cancers (Tables 68 and 72). The significant excess risk of rectal cancer was limited to the period 5 or more years following the uterine cancer. This is consistent with the hypothesis of radiation induction of the rectal carcinoma. Finally, the observed and expected number of second primary rectal cancers was calculated separately for those uterine cancer patients ever treated with radiation and those never treated with radiation. The excess risk was limited to the group which had received radiation.

The excess risk for malignancies of the kidney or ureter in patients with cancer of the uterine corpus has been reported in other studies (BAILAR, 1963; MACMAHON and AUSTIN, 1969; SCHOTTENFELD and BERG, 1971; NEWELL et al., 1974c), but because of the small number of cases the findings from other investigations are not statistically significant. The factor(s) responsible for this association remains unknown.

The increased risk for bladder cancer in patients with cervical cancer has been reported by others (BAILAR, 1963; MORTON and VILLASANTA, 1973; NEWELL et al., 1974c). For cervical cancer patients, malignancies of the oral cavity and pharynx have been reported to occur more often than expected (BAILAR, 1963; SCHOTTENFELD and BERG, 1971; NEWELL et al., 1974c), but the number of cases is small and the results are not statistically significant. Patients with cervical cancer have also been shown to be at increased risk for lung cancer (BAILAR, 1963; SCHOTTENFELD and BERG, 1971; MORTON and VILLASANTA, 1973; NEWELL et al., 1974c). It is interesting that each of these tumors linked with cervical cancer is also strongly correlated with cigarette smoking (LILIENFELD et al., 1956; HAMMOND and HORN, 1958; DOLL and HILL, 1964; HIGGINSON and MUIR, 1973). It may be that heavy cigarette consumption is associated with the demographic subgroup of the female population at high risk of cervical cancer. One might think that bladder cancer following cervical cancer may also be a result of radiotherapy for the cervical lesion. However, the excess risk of bladder cancer was almost as large within the first year following the diagnosis of cervical cancer as it was in the first through fourth years following diagnosis. The excess risk fell off somewhat, 5 or more years after the diagnosis of cervical cancer.

The relationship between prostatic cancer and leukemia is bidirectional. That is, patients with prostatic cancer are at increased risk for leukemia and vice versa. Such evidence is suggestive that a particular oncogenic factor is operating in the development of both neoplasms. However, in a substantial percentage of the patients, both malignancies were not histologically confirmed. Thus, leukemic infiltration of the prostate may have been interpreted clinically as representing prostatic carcinoma. Out of the total of 39 patients with both malignancies, the leukemia was diagnosed prior to the prostatic cancer in 18 individuals (Table 107). The potential bias of asymptomatic prostatic malignancies being first recognized at autopsy examination performed on patients dying with leukemia must also be considered; without the autopsy, the prostatic lesion would have been missed. Furthermore, it may be that patients dying with leukemia come to autopsy more frequently than the general population of deaths. The relationship between prostatic cancer and leukemia has been described in case reports (LYNCH et al., 1966; GUERRIER and PERSKY, 1969), but has yet to be otherwise corroborated in other analytical case-control comparisons.

Also, patients with testicular cancer have an increased risk for developing leukemia. The excess risk appears to be concentrated in the time period beginning 5 years after the diagnosis of the testicular neoplasm. All three patients with leukemia following testicular cancer had both neoplasms verified by microscopic examination. There was only one individual with a testicular malignancy diagnosed after leukemia (Table 107).

If real, the biologic mechanism for this association requires an explanation.

On first inspection, it would appear that the excess risk of malignancies of the eye in breast cancer patients should be listed in category I as being artifactual. This association is based on only five patients and is unsupported by other investigations. Although the eye is a metastatic site for breast cancer, all five patients with this combination of tumors had both malignancies microscopically confirmed. Further analysis revealed that four of the eye tumors were malignant melanomas. The association between malignant melanoma and breast cancer was also noted in a study reporting the experience of the Fox Chase Cancer Center Melanoma Clinic in Philadelphia (VAISMAN et al., 1976). Furthermore, in an investigation of data obtained during the Third National Cancer Survey in the United States, both breast cancer and malignant melanoma showed unexpected positive correlations with alcohol consumption (WILLIAMS, 1976). These relationships remained after controlling for age, race, and smoking status of the cancer patients. WILLIAMS hypothesized that 1) alcohol consumption resulted in a generalized pituitary hypersecretion of several hormones, including prolactin and melanocyte-stimulating hormone, and 2) these hormones may be related to an increased risk of breast cancer and malignant melanoma, respectively. As in the case of meningioma and breast cancer, more detailed analysis by histologic type revealed a previously unexpected association.

The deficiencies of observed-over-expected subsequent primary malignancies for patients with index tumors of the breast and genital organs are listed in Table 93. The deficiency of nervous system malignancies in patients with breast cancer may be related to the fact that the brain is a frequent metastatic site for cancer of the breast. A breast cancer patient presenting with signs or symptoms of an intracranial lesion may be diagnosed as having metastatic disease without benefit of further investigations which might detect an independent primary neoplasm of the brain. The investigation of the Connecticut data, which revealed a significant association between breast cancer and meningioma, included both benign and malignant central nervous system neoplasms (SCHOENBERG et al., 1975). The present study is confined to tumors specified as malignant.

The statistically significant deficit of cervical cancer in patients with endometrial cancer probably illustrates the effect of treatment for the initial cancer. With complete hysterectomy, both the uterine corpus and cervix are removed so that the patient is no longer at risk for developing cancer of the uterine cervix.

The other deficiencies noted in Table 93 remain unexplained.

Table 63. Subsequent multiple primary malignancies in patients with an index malignant tumor of the breast

FIRST PRIMARY SITE - BREAST

| SUBSEQUENT PRIMARY SITES | TOTAL | | | MALES | | | FEMALES | | |
|---|---|---|---|---|---|---|---|---|---|
| | NUMBER OF PERSONS= 18140 PERSON-YRS OF OBSERVATION = 97602.0 | | | NUMBER OF PERSONS= 130 PERSON-YRS OF OBSERVATION = 667.1 | | | NUMBER OF PERSONS= 18010 PERSON-YRS OF OBSERVATION = 96934.9 | | |
| | OBS | EXP | OBS/EXP | OBS | EXP | OBS/EXP | OBS | EXP | OBS/EXP |
| LIP | 2 | 1.12 | 1.79 | 0 | 0.16 | 0.0 | 2 | 0.96 | 2.09 |
| TONGUE | 5 | 2.20 | 2.28 | 2 | 0.12 | 16.39* | 3 | 2.07 | 1.45 |
| SALIVARY GLAND | 2 | 2.14 | 0.93 | 0 | 0.03 | 0.0 | 2 | 2.12 | 0.94 |
| MOUTH | 4 | 3.58 | 1.12 | 0 | 0.16 | 0.0 | 4 | 3.42 | 1.17 |
| PHARYNX | 5 | 3.03 | 1.65 | 1 | 0.15 | 6.83 | 4 | 2.89 | 1.39 |
| ESOPHAGUS | 3 | 4.68 | 0.64 | 0 | 0.27 | 0.0 | 3 | 4.41 | 0.68 |
| STOMACH | 47 | 50.41 | 0.93 | 0 | 1.01 | 0.0 | 47 | 49.40 | 0.95 |
| SMALL INTESTINE | 3 | 2.84 | 1.06 | 0 | 0.03 | 0.0 | 3 | 2.81 | 1.07 |
| COLON | 125 | 106.75 | 1.17 | 0 | 1.12 | 0.0 | 125 | 105.62 | 1.18 |
| RECTUM | 49 | 46.09 | 1.06 | 2 | 0.71 | 2.81 | 47 | 45.38 | 1.04 |
| LIVER & BILIARY PASS | 21 | 22.70 | 0.92 | 0 | 0.22 | 0.0 | 21 | 22.49 | 0.93 |
| PANCREAS | 13 | 22.98 | 0.57* | 1 | 0.36 | 2.75 | 12 | 22.62 | 0.53* |
| NOSE AND SINUSES | 1 | 1.22 | 0.82 | 0 | 0.02 | 0.0 | 1 | 1.20 | 0.84 |
| LARYNX | 1 | 1.69 | 0.59 | 0 | 0.20 | 0.0 | 1 | 1.49 | 0.67 |
| LUNG AND BRONCHUS | 19 | 19.88 | 0.96 | 0 | 1.06 | 0.0 | 19 | 18.82 | 1.01 |
| OTHER RESP | 2 | 0.60 | 3.35 | 0 | 0.02 | 0.0 | 2 | 0.58 | 3.45 |
| BREAST | 597 | 179.69 | 3.32** | 1 | 0.03 | 39.54* | 596 | 179.67 | 3.32** |
| CERVIX UTERI | 51 | 45.87 | 1.11 | 0 | 0.0 | 0.0 | 51 | 45.87 | 1.11 |
| CORPUS UTERI | 71 | 37.52 | 1.89** | 0 | 0.0 | 0.0 | 71 | 37.52 | 1.89** |
| UTERUS,UNSPEC | 23 | 21.29 | 1.08 | 0 | 0.0 | 0.0 | 23 | 21.29 | 1.08 |
| OVARY | 60 | 35.19 | 1.70** | 0 | 0.0 | 0.0 | 60 | 35.19 | 1.70** |
| OTHER FEMALE GENITAL | 6 | 7.67 | 0.78 | 0 | 0.0 | 0.0 | 6 | 7.67 | 0.78 |
| PROSTATE | 4 | 1.92 | 2.08 | 4 | 1.92 | 2.08 | 0 | 0.0 | 0.0 |
| TESTIS | 0 | 0.02 | 0.0 | 0 | 0.02 | 0.0 | 0 | 0.0 | 0.0 |
| OTHER MALE GENITAL | 0 | 0.04 | 0.0 | 0 | 0.04 | 0.0 | 0 | 0.0 | 0.0 |
| KIDNEY AND URETER | 6 | 11.12 | 0.54 | 0 | 0.19 | 0.0 | 6 | 10.92 | 0.55 |
| BLADDER | 25 | 21.98 | 1.14 | 0 | 0.70 | 0.0 | 25 | 21.28 | 1.17 |
| MELANOMA OF SKIN | 8 | 5.76 | 1.39 | 0 | 0.05 | 0.0 | 8 | 5.71 | 1.40 |
| EYE | 5 | 1.48 | 3.37* | 0 | 0.02 | 0.0 | 5 | 1.47 | 3.41* |
| NERVOUS SYSTEM | 1 | 7.58 | 0.13** | 0 | 0.06 | 0.0 | 1 | 7.52 | 0.13** |
| THYROID | 6 | 5.65 | 1.06 | 0 | 0.02 | 0.0 | 6 | 5.63 | 1.07 |
| BONE | 2 | 2.08 | 0.96 | 0 | 0.03 | 0.0 | 2 | 2.06 | 0.97 |
| SOFT TISSUE | 15 | 4.53 | 3.31** | 2 | 0.06 | 36.03** | 13 | 4.47 | 2.91** |
| LYMPHOMAS & MYELOMA | 14 | 19.10 | 0.73 | 0 | 0.23 | 0.0 | 14 | 18.87 | 0.74 |
| LEUKEMIAS | 15 | 17.21 | 0.87 | 2 | 0.27 | 7.46 | 13 | 16.94 | 0.77 |
| OTHER SITES | 19 | 42.33 | 0.45** | 0 | 0.49 | 0.0 | 19 | 41.85 | 0.45** |
| TOTAL | 1230 | 759.93 | 1.62** | 15 | 9.74 | 1.54 | 1215 | 750.19 | 1.62** |

Table 64. Subsequent primary sites with excesses

FIRST PRIMARY SITE - BREAST

| SUBSEQUENT PRIMARY SITES | TOTAL<br>NUMBER OF PERSONS= 18140<br>PERSON-YRS OF OBSERVATION= 97602.1 | | | YEARS < 1<br>NUMBER OF PERSONS= 18140<br>PERSON-YRS OF OBSERVATION= 16502.5 | | | YEARS 1-5<br>NUMBER OF PERSONS= 14983<br>PERSON-YRS OF OBSERVATION= 40507.4 | | | YEARS > 5<br>NUMBER OF PERSONS= 6734<br>PERSON-YRS OF OBSERVATION= 40592.2 | | |
|---|---|---|---|---|---|---|---|---|---|---|---|---|
| | OBS | EXP | OBS/EXP | OBS | EXP | OBS/EXP | OBS | EXP | OBS/EXP | OBS | EXP | OBS/EXP |
| TONGUE | 5 | 2.20 | 2.28 | 0 | 0.32 | 0.0 | 3 | 0.85 | 3.52 | 2 | 1.03 | 1.95 |
| COLON | 125 | 106.75 | 1.17 | 10 | 14.94 | 0.67 | 38 | 40.09 | 0.95 | 77 | 51.72 | 1.49** |
| BREAST | 597 | 179.69 | 3.32** | 109 | 27.30 | 3.99** | 262 | 70.65 | 3.71** | 226 | 81.75 | 2.76** |
| CORPUS UTERI | 71 | 37.52 | 1.89** | 10 | 5.43 | 1.84 | 30 | 14.37 | 2.09** | 31 | 17.72 | 1.75** |
| OVARY | 60 | 35.19 | 1.70** | 7 | 5.42 | 1.29 | 18 | 13.95 | 1.29 | 35 | 15.82 | 2.21** |
| BLADDER | 25 | 21.98 | 1.14 | 2 | 3.02 | 0.66 | 15 | 8.16 | 1.84* | 8 | 10.80 | 0.74 |
| EYE | 5 | 1.48 | 3.37* | 0 | 0.22 | 0.0 | 3 | 0.58 | 5.20* | 2 | 0.69 | 2.92 |
| SOFT TISSUE | 15 | 4.53 | 3.31** | 3 | 0.65 | 4.61 | 4 | 1.71 | 2.34 | 8 | 2.17 | 3.69** |

Table 65. Subsequent primary sites with deficiencies

FIRST PRIMARY SITE - BREAST

| SUBSEQUENT PRIMARY SITES | TOTAL<br>NUMBER OF PERSONS= 18140<br>PERSON-YRS OF OBSERVATION= 97602.1 | | | YEARS < 1<br>NUMBER OF PERSONS= 18140<br>PERSON-YRS OF OBSERVATION= 16502.5 | | | YEARS 1-5<br>NUMBER OF PERSONS= 14983<br>PERSON-YRS OF OBSERVATION= 40507.4 | | | YEARS > 5<br>NUMBER OF PERSONS= 6734<br>PERSON-YRS OF OBSERVATION= 40592.2 | | |
|---|---|---|---|---|---|---|---|---|---|---|---|---|
| | OBS | EXP | OBS/EXP | OBS | EXP | OBS/EXP | OBS | EXP | OBS/EXP | OBS | EXP | OBS/EXP |
| PANCREAS | 13 | 22.98 | 0.57* | 4 | 3.21 | 1.25 | 7 | 8.59 | 0.81 | 2 | 11.18 | 0.18** |
| NERVOUS SYSTEM | 1 | 7.58 | 0.13** | 0 | 1.23 | 0.0 | 1 | 3.08 | 0.32 | 0 | 3.27 | 0.0 |
| OTHER SITES | 19 | 42.33 | 0.45** | 0 | 5.78 | 0.0 | 6 | 15.65 | 0.38* | 13 | 20.90 | 0.62 |

Table 66. Histologic confirmation of multiple primary malignancies

FIRST PRIMARY SITE - BREAST

| Subsequent primary site | Both tumors microscopically confirmed | | Only 1st tumor microscopically confirmed | | Only 2nd tumor microscopically confirmed | | Neither tumor microscopically confirmed | |
|---|---|---|---|---|---|---|---|---|
| | No. | % | No. | % | No. | % | No. | % |
| TONGUE | 3 | 60.0 | 2 | 40.0 | 0 | 0.0 | 0 | 0.0 |
| COLON | 100 | 80.0 | 18 | 14.4 | 6 | 4.8 | 1 | 0.8 |
| BREAST | 543 | 91.0 | 23 | 3.9 | 27 | 4.5 | 4 | 0.7 |
| CORPUS UTERI | 65 | 91.5 | 2 | 2.8 | 3 | 4.2 | 1 | 1.4 |
| OVARY | 55 | 91.7 | 3 | 5.0 | 2 | 3.3 | 0 | 0.0 |
| BLADDER | 18 | 72.0 | 6 | 24.0 | 0 | 0.0 | 1 | 4.0 |
| EYE | 5 | 100.0 | 0 | 0.0 | 0 | 0.0 | 0 | 0.0 |
| SOFT TISSUE | 14 | 93.3 | 1 | 6.7 | 0 | 0.0 | 0 | 0.0 |

Table 67. Subsequent multiple primary malignancies in patients with an index malignant tumor of the cervix uteri

FIRST PRIMARY SITE - CERVIX UTERI

| SUBSEQUENT PRIMARY SITES | TOTAL NUMBER OF PERSONS= 7456 PERSON-YRS OF OBSERVATION = 41475.2 | | | FEMALES NUMBER OF PERSONS= 7456 PERSON-YRS OF OBSERVATION = 41475.2 | | |
|---|---|---|---|---|---|---|
| | OBS | EXP | OBS/EXP | OBS | EXP | OBS/EXP |
| LIP | 1 | 0.25 | 3.93 | 1 | 0.25 | 3.93 |
| TONGUE | 0 | 0.64 | 0.0 | 0 | 0.64 | 0.0 |
| SALIVARY GLAND | 1 | 0.64 | 1.56 | 1 | 0.64 | 1.56 |
| MOUTH | 2 | 0.94 | 2.14 | 2 | 0.94 | 2.14 |
| PHARYNX | 4 | 0.94 | 4.24* | 4 | 0.94 | 4.24* |
| ESOPHAGUS | 1 | 1.17 | 0.86 | 1 | 1.17 | 0.86 |
| STOMACH | 17 | 12.04 | 1.41 | 17 | 12.04 | 1.41 |
| SMALL INTESTINE | 0 | 0.79 | 0.0 | 0 | 0.79 | 0.0 |
| COLON | 28 | 28.46 | 0.98 | 28 | 28.46 | 0.98 |
| RECTUM | 24 | 13.05 | 1.84** | 24 | 13.05 | 1.84** |
| LIVER & BILIARY PASS | 1 | 5.58 | 0.18* | 1 | 5.58 | 0.18* |
| PANCREAS | 4 | 5.90 | 0.68 | 4 | 5.90 | 0.68 |
| NOSE AND SINUSES | 1 | 0.39 | 2.59 | 1 | 0.39 | 2.59 |
| LARYNX | 2 | 0.58 | 3.47 | 2 | 0.58 | 3.47 |
| LUNG AND BRONCHUS | 25 | 5.72 | 4.37** | 25 | 5.72 | 4.37** |
| OTHER RESP | 0 | 0.20 | 0.0 | 0 | 0.20 | 0.0 |
| BREAST | 52 | 60.63 | 0.86 | 52 | 60.63 | 0.86 |
| CERVIX UTERI | 0 | 20.86 | 0.0 | 0 | 20.86 | 0.0 |
| CORPUS UTERI | 15 | 13.41 | 1.12 | 15 | 13.41 | 1.12 |
| UTERUS,UNSPEC | 2 | 6.66 | 0.30 | 2 | 6.66 | 0.30 |
| OVARY | 17 | 12.80 | 1.33 | 17 | 12.80 | 1.33 |
| OTHER FEMALE GENITAL | 11 | 2.06 | 5.35** | 11 | 2.06 | 5.35** |
| PROSTATE | 0 | 0.0 | 0.0 | 0 | 0.0 | 0.0 |
| TESTIS | 0 | 0.0 | 0.0 | 0 | 0.0 | 0.0 |
| OTHER MALE GENITAL | 0 | 0.0 | 0.0 | 0 | 0.0 | 0.0 |
| KIDNEY AND URETER | 7 | 3.26 | 2.15 | 7 | 3.26 | 2.15 |
| BLADDER | 22 | 5.31 | 4.14** | 22 | 5.31 | 4.14** |
| MELANOMA OF SKIN | 1 | 2.19 | 0.46 | 1 | 2.19 | 0.46 |
| EYE | 1 | 0.44 | 2.26 | 1 | 0.44 | 2.26 |
| NERVOUS SYSTEM | 1 | 3.04 | 0.33 | 1 | 3.04 | 0.33 |
| THYROID | 0 | 1.97 | 0.0 | 0 | 1.97 | 0.0 |
| BONE | 1 | 0.64 | 1.57 | 1 | 0.64 | 1.57 |
| SOFT TISSUE | 4 | 1.60 | 2.50 | 4 | 1.60 | 2.50 |
| LYMPHOMAS & MYELOMA | 9 | 6.31 | 1.43 | 9 | 6.31 | 1.43 |
| LEUKEMIAS | 7 | 4.97 | 1.41 | 7 | 4.97 | 1.41 |
| OTHER SITES | 18 | 11.11 | 1.62 | 18 | 11.11 | 1.62 |
| TOTAL | 279 | 234.53 | 1.19** | 279 | 234.53 | 1.19** |

Table 68. Subsequent primary sites with excesses

FIRST PRIMARY SITE - CERVIX UTERI

| SUBSEQUENT PRIMARY SITES | TOTAL | | | YEARS < 1 | | | YEARS 1-5 | | | YEARS > 5 | | |
|---|---|---|---|---|---|---|---|---|---|---|---|---|
| | NUMBER OF PERSONS= 7456 PERSON-YRS OF OBSERVATION= 41475.2 | | | NUMBER OF PERSONS= 7456 PERSON-YRS OF OBSERVATION= 6672.3 | | | NUMBER OF PERSONS= 5893 PERSON-YRS OF OBSERVATION= 15952.2 | | | NUMBER OF PERSONS= 2861 PERSON-YRS OF OBSERVATION= 18850.7 | | |
| | OBS | EXP | OBS/EXP | OBS | EXP | OBS/EXP | OBS | EXP | OBS/EXP | OBS | EXP | OBS/EXP |
| PHARYNX | 4 | 0.94 | 4.24* | 0 | 0.11 | 0.0 | 1 | 0.31 | 3.27 | 3 | 0.52 | 5.72* |
| RECTUM | 24 | 13.05 | 1.84** | 2 | 1.59 | 1.26 | 7 | 4.11 | 1.70 | 15 | 7.35 | 2.04* |
| LUNG AND BRONCHUS | 25 | 5.72 | 4.37** | 0 | 0.65 | 0.0 | 12 | 1.77 | 6.77** | 13 | 3.30 | 3.94** |
| OTHER FEMALE GENITAL | 11 | 2.06 | 5.35** | 0 | 0.25 | 0.0 | 6 | 0.65 | 9.23** | 5 | 1.16 | 4.32* |
| BLADDER | 22 | 5.31 | 4.14** | 3 | 0.61 | 4.91* | 11 | 1.61 | 6.85** | 8 | 3.09 | 2.59* |
| OTHER SITES | 18 | 11.11 | 1.62 | 2 | 1.26 | 1.58 | 8 | 3.37 | 2.38* | 8 | 6.48 | 1.23 |

Table 69. Subsequent primary sites with deficiencies

FIRST PRIMARY SITE - CERVIX UTERI

| SUBSEQUENT PRIMARY SITES | TOTAL | | | YEARS < 1 | | | YEARS 1-5 | | | YEARS > 5 | | |
|---|---|---|---|---|---|---|---|---|---|---|---|---|
| | NUMBER OF PERSONS= 7456 PERSON-YRS OF OBSERVATION= 41475.2 | | | NUMBER OF PERSONS= 7456 PERSON-YRS OF OBSERVATION= 6672.3 | | | NUMBER OF PERSONS= 5893 PERSON-YRS OF OBSERVATION= 15952.2 | | | NUMBER OF PERSONS= 2861 PERSON-YRS OF OBSERVATION= 18850.7 | | |
| | OBS | EXP | OBS/EXP | OBS | EXP | OBS/EXP | OBS | EXP | OBS/EXP | OBS | EXP | OBS/EXP |
| LIVER & BILIARY PASS | 1 | 5.58 | 0.18* | 0 | 0.70 | 0.0 | 0 | 1.74 | 0.0 | 1 | 3.13 | 0.32 |

Table 70. Histologic confirmation of multiple primary malignancies

FIRST PRIMARY SITE - CERVIX UTERI

| Subsequent primary site | Both tumors microscopically confirmed | | Only 1st tumor microscopically confirmed | | Only 2nd tumor microscopically confirmed | | Neither tumor microscopically confirmed | |
|---|---|---|---|---|---|---|---|---|
| | No. | % | No. | % | No. | % | No. | % |
| PHARYNX | 4 | 100.0 | 0 | 0.0 | 0 | 0.0 | 0 | 0.0 |
| RECTUM | 17 | 70.8 | 7 | 29.2 | 0 | 0.0 | 0 | 0.0 |
| LUNG AND BRONCHUS | 19 | 76.0 | 5 | 20.0 | 1 | 4.0 | 0 | 0.0 |
| OTHER FEMALE GENITAL | 10 | 90.9 | 0 | 0.0 | 0 | 0.0 | 1 | 9.1 |
| BLADDER | 14 | 63.6 | 5 | 22.7 | 2 | 9.1 | 1 | 4.5 |
| OTHER SITES | 15 | 83.3 | 3 | 16.7 | 0 | 0.0 | 0 | 0.0 |

Table 71. Subsequent multiple primary malignancies in patients with an index malignant tumor of the corpus uteri

FIRST PRIMARY SITE - CORPUS UTERI

| SUBSEQUENT PRIMARY SITES | TOTAL: NUMBER OF PERSONS= 3958, PERSON-YRS OF OBSERVATION = 24359.0 | | | FEMALES: NUMBER OF PERSONS= 3958, PERSON-YRS OF OBSERVATION = 24359.0 | | |
|---|---|---|---|---|---|---|
| | OBS | EXP | OBS/EXP | OBS | EXP | OBS/EXP |
| LIP | 1 | 0.24 | 4.11 | 1 | 0.24 | 4.11 |
| TONGUE | 0 | 0.54 | 0.0 | 0 | 0.54 | 0.0 |
| SALIVARY GLAND | 1 | 0.53 | 1.89 | 1 | 0.53 | 1.89 |
| MOUTH | 1 | 0.84 | 1.19 | 1 | 0.84 | 1.19 |
| PHARYNX | 0 | 0.76 | 0.0 | 0 | 0.76 | 0.0 |
| ESOPHAGUS | 1 | 1.09 | 0.92 | 1 | 1.09 | 0.92 |
| STOMACH | 5 | 11.86 | 0.42* | 5 | 11.86 | 0.42* |
| SMALL INTESTINE | 1 | 0.72 | 1.39 | 1 | 0.72 | 1.39 |
| COLON | 40 | 27.39 | 1.46* | 40 | 27.39 | 1.46* |
| RECTUM | 21 | 11.97 | 1.75* | 21 | 11.97 | 1.75* |
| LIVER & BILIARY PASS | 4 | 5.64 | 0.71 | 4 | 5.64 | 0.71 |
| PANCREAS | 6 | 5.95 | 1.01 | 6 | 5.95 | 1.01 |
| NOSE AND SINUSES | 0 | 0.31 | 0.0 | 0 | 0.31 | 0.0 |
| LARYNX | 0 | 0.40 | 0.0 | 0 | 0.40 | 0.0 |
| LUNG AND BRONCHUS | 6 | 5.08 | 1.18 | 6 | 5.08 | 1.18 |
| OTHER RESP | 0 | 0.14 | 0.0 | 0 | 0.14 | 0.0 |
| BREAST | 66 | 46.07 | 1.43** | 66 | 46.07 | 1.43** |
| CERVIX UTERI | 4 | 11.70 | 0.34* | 4 | 11.70 | 0.34* |
| CORPUS UTERI | 0 | 10.76 | 0.0 | 0 | 10.76 | 0.0 |
| UTERUS,UNSPEC | 0 | 5.29 | 0.0 | 0 | 5.29 | 0.0 |
| OVARY | 9 | 9.56 | 0.94 | 9 | 9.56 | 0.94 |
| OTHER FEMALE GENITAL | 8 | 1.94 | 4.13** | 8 | 1.94 | 4.13** |
| PROSTATE | 0 | 0.0 | 0.0 | 0 | 0.0 | 0.0 |
| TESTIS | 0 | 0.0 | 0.0 | 0 | 0.0 | 0.0 |
| OTHER MALE GENITAL | 0 | 0.0 | 0.0 | 0 | 0.0 | 0.0 |
| KIDNEY AND URETER | 8 | 2.94 | 2.72* | 8 | 2.94 | 2.72* |
| BLADDER | 7 | 5.30 | 1.32 | 7 | 5.30 | 1.32 |
| MELANOMA OF SKIN | 1 | 1.55 | 0.65 | 1 | 1.55 | 0.65 |
| EYE | 2 | 0.38 | 5.30 | 2 | 0.38 | 5.30 |
| NERVOUS SYSTEM | 1 | 2.04 | 0.49 | 1 | 2.04 | 0.49 |
| THYROID | 2 | 1.41 | 1.42 | 2 | 1.41 | 1.42 |
| BONE | 0 | 0.54 | 0.0 | 0 | 0.54 | 0.0 |
| SOFT TISSUE | 2 | 1.25 | 1.60 | 2 | 1.25 | 1.60 |
| LYMPHOMAS & MYELOMA | 9 | 5.34 | 1.68 | 9 | 5.34 | 1.68 |
| LEUKEMIAS | 7 | 4.65 | 1.51 | 7 | 4.65 | 1.51 |
| OTHER SITES | 8 | 10.76 | 0.74 | 8 | 10.76 | 0.74 |
| TOTAL | 221 | 194.94 | 1.13 | 221 | 194.94 | 1.13 |

Table 72. Subsequent primary sites with excesses

FIRST PRIMARY SITE - CORPUS UTERI

| | TOTAL | | | YEARS < 1 | | | YEARS 1-5 | | | YEARS > 5 | | |
|---|---|---|---|---|---|---|---|---|---|---|---|---|
| | NUMBER OF PERSONS= 3958 PERSON-YRS OF OBSERVATION= 24359.0 | | | NUMBER OF PERSONS= 3958 PERSON-YRS OF OBSERVATION= 3531.2 | | | NUMBER OF PERSONS= 3203 PERSON-YRS OF OBSERVATION= 9374.5 | | | NUMBER OF PERSONS= 1744 PERSON-YRS OF OBSERVATION= 11453.3 | | |
| SUBSEQUENT PRIMARY SITES | OBS | EXP | OBS/EXP | OBS | EXP | OBS/EXP | OBS | EXP | OBS/EXP | OBS | EXP | OBS/EXP |
| COLON | 40 | 27.39 | 1.46* | 0 | 3.31 | 0.0 | 17 | 9.22 | 1.84* | 23 | 14.86 | 1.55 |
| RECTUM | 21 | 11.97 | 1.75* | 0 | 1.51 | 0.0 | 7 | 4.17 | 1.68 | 14 | 6.29 | 2.23* |
| BREAST | 66 | 46.07 | 1.43** | 6 | 6.12 | 0.98 | 30 | 16.69 | 1.80** | 30 | 23.26 | 1.29 |
| OVARY | 9 | 9.56 | 0.94 | 6 | 1.28 | 4.68** | 0 | 3.50 | 0.0 | 3 | 4.77 | 0.63 |
| OTHER FEMALE GENITAL | 8 | 1.94 | 4.13** | 1 | 0.24 | 4.25 | 1 | 0.66 | 1.52 | 6 | 1.04 | 5.75** |
| KIDNEY AND URETER | 8 | 2.94 | 2.72* | 1 | 0.36 | 2.79 | 3 | 1.01 | 2.97 | 4 | 1.58 | 2.54 |

Table 73. Subsequent primary sites with deficiencies

FIRST PRIMARY SITE - CORPUS UTERI

| | TOTAL | | | YEARS < 1 | | | YEARS 1-5 | | | YEARS > 5 | | |
|---|---|---|---|---|---|---|---|---|---|---|---|---|
| | NUMBER OF PERSONS= 3958 PERSON-YRS OF OBSERVATION= 24359.0 | | | NUMBER OF PERSONS= 3958 PERSON-YRS OF OBSERVATION= 3531.2 | | | NUMBER OF PERSONS= 3203 PERSON-YRS OF OBSERVATION= 9374.5 | | | NUMBER OF PERSONS= 1744 PERSON-YRS OF OBSERVATION= 11453.3 | | |
| SUBSEQUENT PRIMARY SITES | OBS | EXP | OBS/EXP | OBS | EXP | OBS/EXP | OBS | EXP | OBS/EXP | OBS | EXP | OBS/EXP |
| STOMACH | 5 | 11.86 | 0.42* | 1 | 1.55 | 0.65 | 2 | 4.12 | 0.49 | 2 | 6.19 | 0.32 |
| CERVIX UTERI | 4 | 11.70 | 0.34* | 1 | 1.73 | 0.58 | 2 | 4.58 | 0.44 | 1 | 5.38 | 0.19 |

Table 74. Histologic confirmation of multiple primary malignancies

FIRST PRIMARY SITE - CORPUS UTERI

| Subsequent primary site | Both tumors microscopically confirmed | | Only 1st tumor microscopically confirmed | | Only 2nd tumor microscopically confirmed | | Neither tumor microscopically confirmed | |
|---|---|---|---|---|---|---|---|---|
| | No. | % | No. | % | No. | % | No. | % |
| COLON | 37 | 92.5 | 3 | 7.5 | 0 | 0.0 | 0 | 0.0 |
| RECTUM | 19 | 90.5 | 2 | 9.5 | 0 | 0.0 | 0 | 0.0 |
| BREAST | 58 | 87.9 | 6 | 9.1 | 2 | 3.0 | 0 | 0.0 |
| OVARY | 8 | 88.9 | 0 | 0.0 | 1 | 11.1 | 0 | 0.0 |
| OTHER FEMALE GENITAL | 7 | 87.5 | 1 | 12.5 | 0 | 0.0 | 0 | 0.0 |
| KIDNEY AND URETER | 7 | 87.5 | 1 | 12.5 | 0 | 0.0 | 0 | 0.0 |

Table 75. Subsequent multiple primary malignancies in patients with an index malignant tumor of the uterus, unspecified

FIRST PRIMARY SITE - UTERUS UNSPECIFIED

| SUBSEQUENT PRIMARY SITES | TOTAL<br>NUMBER OF PERSONS= 1568<br>PERSON-YRS OF OBSERVATION = 10501.4 | | | FEMALES<br>NUMBER OF PERSONS= 1568<br>PERSON-YRS OF OBSERVATION = 10501.4 | | |
|---|---|---|---|---|---|---|
| | OBS | EXP | OBS/EXP | OBS | EXP | OBS/EXP |
| LIP | 0 | 0.11 | 0.0 | 0 | 0.11 | 0.0 |
| TONGUE | 0 | 0.23 | 0.0 | 0 | 0.23 | 0.0 |
| SALIVARY GLAND | 0 | 0.23 | 0.0 | 0 | 0.23 | 0.0 |
| MOUTH | 0 | 0.35 | 0.0 | 0 | 0.35 | 0.0 |
| PHARYNX | 2 | 0.32 | 6.27 | 2 | 0.32 | 6.27 |
| ESOPHAGUS | 0 | 0.47 | 0.0 | 0 | 0.47 | 0.0 |
| STOMACH | 6 | 5.17 | 1.16 | 6 | 5.17 | 1.16 |
| SMALL INTESTINE | 0 | 0.31 | 0.0 | 0 | 0.31 | 0.0 |
| COLON | 14 | 11.62 | 1.20 | 14 | 11.62 | 1.20 |
| RECTUM | 10 | 5.15 | 1.94 | 10 | 5.15 | 1.94 |
| LIVER & BILIARY PASS | 0 | 2.45 | 0.0 | 0 | 2.45 | 0.0 |
| PANCREAS | 2 | 2.50 | 0.80 | 2 | 2.50 | 0.80 |
| NOSE AND SINUSES | 0 | 0.13 | 0.0 | 0 | 0.13 | 0.0 |
| LARYNX | 0 | 0.16 | 0.0 | 0 | 0.16 | 0.0 |
| LUNG AND BRONCHUS | 3 | 2.09 | 1.43 | 3 | 2.09 | 1.43 |
| OTHER RESP | 0 | 0.06 | 0.0 | 0 | 0.06 | 0.0 |
| BREAST | 20 | 19.56 | 1.02 | 20 | 19.56 | 1.02 |
| CERVIX UTERI | 2 | 5.04 | 0.40 | 2 | 5.04 | 0.40 |
| CORPUS UTERI | 0 | 4.49 | 0.0 | 0 | 4.49 | 0.0 |
| UTERUS,UNSPEC | 0 | 2.42 | 0.0 | 0 | 2.42 | 0.0 |
| OVARY | 5 | 4.08 | 1.23 | 5 | 4.08 | 1.23 |
| OTHER FEMALE GENITAL | 2 | 0.83 | 2.42 | 2 | 0.83 | 2.42 |
| PROSTATE | 0 | 0.0 | 0.0 | 0 | 0.0 | 0.0 |
| TESTIS | 0 | 0.0 | 0.0 | 0 | 0.0 | 0.0 |
| OTHER MALE GENITAL | 0 | 0.0 | 0.0 | 0 | 0.0 | 0.0 |
| KIDNEY AND URETER | 0 | 1.25 | 0.0 | 0 | 1.25 | 0.0 |
| BLADDER | 4 | 2.24 | 1.79 | 4 | 2.24 | 1.79 |
| MELANOMA OF SKIN | 1 | 0.63 | 1.58 | 1 | 0.63 | 1.58 |
| EYE | 0 | 0.17 | 0.0 | 0 | 0.17 | 0.0 |
| NERVOUS SYSTEM | 0 | 0.88 | 0.0 | 0 | 0.88 | 0.0 |
| THYROID | 2 | 0.58 | 3.42 | 2 | 0.58 | 3.42 |
| BONE | 0 | 0.24 | 0.0 | 0 | 0.24 | 0.0 |
| SOFT TISSUE | 0 | 0.51 | 0.0 | 0 | 0.51 | 0.0 |
| LYMPHOMAS & MYELOMA | 1 | 2.22 | 0.45 | 1 | 2.22 | 0.45 |
| LEUKEMIAS | 1 | 1.96 | 0.51 | 1 | 1.96 | 0.51 |
| OTHER SITES | 4 | 4.55 | 0.88 | 4 | 4.55 | 0.88 |
| TOTAL | 79 | 82.99 | 0.95 | 79 | 82.99 | 0.95 |

Table 76. Subsequent multiple primary malignancies in patients with an index malignant tumor of the ovary

FIRST PRIMARY SITE - OVARY

| SUBSEQUENT PRIMARY SITES | TOTAL<br>NUMBER OF PERSONS= 3571<br>PERSON-YRS OF OBSERVATION = 11839.2 | | | FEMALES<br>NUMBER OF PERSONS= 3571<br>PERSON-YRS OF OBSERVATION = 11839.2 | | |
|---|---|---|---|---|---|---|
| | OBS | EXP | OBS/EXP | OBS | EXP | OBS/EXP |
| LIP | 0 | 0.08 | 0.0 | 0 | 0.08 | 0.0 |
| TONGUE | 0 | 0.20 | 0.0 | 0 | 0.20 | 0.0 |
| SALIVARY GLAND | 1 | 0.20 | 5.09 | 1 | 0.20 | 5.09 |
| MOUTH | 0 | 0.29 | 0.0 | 0 | 0.29 | 0.0 |
| PHARYNX | 0 | 0.28 | 0.0 | 0 | 0.28 | 0.0 |
| ESOPHAGUS | 0 | 0.37 | 0.0 | 0 | 0.37 | 0.0 |
| STOMACH | 4 | 3.91 | 1.02 | 4 | 3.91 | 1.02 |
| SMALL INTESTINE | 0 | 0.25 | 0.0 | 0 | 0.25 | 0.0 |
| COLON | 19 | 8.99 | 2.11** | 19 | 8.99 | 2.11** |
| RECTUM | 5 | 4.09 | 1.22 | 5 | 4.09 | 1.22 |
| LIVER & BILIARY PASS | 4 | 1.83 | 2.19 | 4 | 1.83 | 2.19 |
| PANCREAS | 1 | 1.90 | 0.53 | 1 | 1.90 | 0.53 |
| NOSE AND SINUSES | 0 | 0.12 | 0.0 | 0 | 0.12 | 0.0 |
| LARYNX | 0 | 0.16 | 0.0 | 0 | 0.16 | 0.0 |
| LUNG AND BRONCHUS | 4 | 1.75 | 2.29 | 4 | 1.75 | 2.29 |
| OTHER RESP | 0 | 0.06 | 0.0 | 0 | 0.06 | 0.0 |
| BREAST | 25 | 17.91 | 1.40 | 25 | 17.91 | 1.40 |
| CERVIX UTERI | 8 | 5.57 | 1.44 | 8 | 5.57 | 1.44 |
| CORPUS UTERI | 10 | 3.97 | 2.52* | 10 | 3.97 | 2.52* |
| UTERUS,UNSPEC | 1 | 2.03 | 0.49 | 1 | 2.03 | 0.49 |
| OVARY | 6 | 3.76 | 1.60 | 6 | 3.76 | 1.60 |
| OTHER FEMALE GENITAL | 1 | 0.65 | 1.55 | 1 | 0.65 | 1.55 |
| PROSTATE | 0 | 0.0 | 0.0 | 0 | 0.0 | 0.0 |
| TESTIS | 0 | 0.0 | 0.0 | 0 | 0.0 | 0.0 |
| OTHER MALE GENITAL | 0 | 0.0 | 0.0 | 0 | 0.0 | 0.0 |
| KIDNEY AND URETER | 2 | 1.01 | 1.98 | 2 | 1.01 | 1.98 |
| BLADDER | 4 | 1.70 | 2.35 | 4 | 1.70 | 2.35 |
| MELANOMA OF SKIN | 1 | 0.62 | 1.61 | 1 | 0.62 | 1.61 |
| EYE | 0 | 0.14 | 0.0 | 0 | 0.14 | 0.0 |
| NERVOUS SYSTEM | 2 | 0.88 | 2.28 | 2 | 0.88 | 2.28 |
| THYROID | 1 | 0.57 | 1.77 | 1 | 0.57 | 1.77 |
| BONE | 0 | 0.19 | 0.0 | 0 | 0.19 | 0.0 |
| SOFT TISSUE | 1 | 0.47 | 2.14 | 1 | 0.47 | 2.14 |
| LYMPHOMAS & MYELOMA | 3 | 1.90 | 1.58 | 3 | 1.90 | 1.58 |
| LEUKEMIAS | 1 | 1.55 | 0.65 | 1 | 1.55 | 0.65 |
| OTHER SITES | 5 | 3.52 | 1.42 | 5 | 3.52 | 1.42 |
| TOTAL | 109 | 70.88 | 1.54** | 109 | 70.88 | 1.54** |

Table 77. Subsequent primary sites with excesses

FIRST PRIMARY SITE - OVARY

| SUBSEQUENT PRIMARY SITES | TOTAL<br>NUMBER OF PERSONS= 3571<br>PERSON-YRS OF OBSERVATION= 11839.2 | | | YEARS < 1<br>NUMBER OF PERSONS= 3571<br>PERSON-YRS OF OBSERVATION= 2530.6 | | | YEARS 1-5<br>NUMBER OF PERSONS= 1848<br>PERSON-YRS OF OBSERVATION= 4284.4 | | | YEARS > 5<br>NUMBER OF PERSONS= 697<br>PERSON-YRS OF OBSERVATION= 5024.2 | | |
|---|---|---|---|---|---|---|---|---|---|---|---|---|
| | OBS | EXP | OBS/EXP | OBS | EXP | OBS/EXP | OBS | EXP | OBS/EXP | OBS | EXP | OBS/EXP |
| COLON | 19 | 8.99 | 2.11** | 6 | 1.78 | 3.37* | 7 | 2.82 | 2.48 | 6 | 4.39 | 1.37 |
| CORPUS UTERI | 10 | 3.97 | 2.52* | 3 | 0.78 | 3.83 | 3 | 1.30 | 2.31 | 4 | 1.88 | 2.12 |

Table 78. Histologic confirmation of multiple primary malignancies

FIRST PRIMARY SITE - OVARY

| Subsequent primary site | Both tumors microscopically confirmed | | Only 1st tumor microscopically confirmed | | Only 2nd tumor microscopically confirmed | | Neither tumor microscopically confirmed | |
|---|---|---|---|---|---|---|---|---|
| | No. | % | No. | % | No. | % | No. | % |
| COLON | 17 | 89.5 | 2 | 10.5 | 0 | 0.0 | 0 | 0.0 |
| CORPUS UTERI | 9 | 90.0 | 1 | 10.0 | 0 | 0.0 | 0 | 0.0 |

Table 79. Subsequent multiple primary malignancies in patients with an index malignant tumor of other and unspecified female genital organs

FIRST PRIMARY SITE - OTHER AND UNSPECIFIED FEMALE GENITAL ORGANS

| SUBSEQUENT PRIMARY SITES | TOTAL<br>NUMBER OF PERSONS= 852<br>PERSON-YRS OF OBSERVATION = 3946.0 | | | FEMALES<br>NUMBER OF PERSONS= 852<br>PERSON-YRS OF OBSERVATION = 3946.0 | | |
|---|---|---|---|---|---|---|
| | OBS | EXP | OBS/EXP | OBS | EXP | OBS/EXP |
| LIP | 0 | 0.05 | 0.0 | 0 | 0.05 | 0.0 |
| TONGUE | 0 | 0.09 | 0.0 | 0 | 0.09 | 0.0 |
| SALIVARY GLAND | 0 | 0.09 | 0.0 | 0 | 0.09 | 0.0 |
| MOUTH | 0 | 0.16 | 0.0 | 0 | 0.16 | 0.0 |
| PHARYNX | 0 | 0.12 | 0.0 | 0 | 0.12 | 0.0 |
| ESOPHAGUS | 2 | 0.20 | 10.00* | 2 | 0.20 | 10.00* |
| STOMACH | 0 | 2.35 | 0.0 | 0 | 2.35 | 0.0 |
| SMALL INTESTINE | 0 | 0.13 | 0.0 | 0 | 0.13 | 0.0 |
| COLON | 3 | 4.82 | 0.62 | 3 | 4.82 | 0.62 |
| RECTUM | 1 | 2.00 | 0.50 | 1 | 2.00 | 0.50 |
| LIVER & BILIARY PASS | 1 | 1.05 | 0.96 | 1 | 1.05 | 0.96 |
| PANCREAS | 0 | 1.03 | 0.0 | 0 | 1.03 | 0.0 |
| NOSE AND SINUSES | 0 | 0.05 | 0.0 | 0 | 0.05 | 0.0 |
| LARYNX | 0 | 0.06 | 0.0 | 0 | 0.06 | 0.0 |
| LUNG AND BRONCHUS | 0 | 0.81 | 0.0 | 0 | 0.81 | 0.0 |
| OTHER RESP | 0 | 0.02 | 0.0 | 0 | 0.02 | 0.0 |
| BREAST | 4 | 7.51 | 0.53 | 4 | 7.51 | 0.53 |
| CERVIX UTERI | 5 | 1.76 | 2.84 | 5 | 1.76 | 2.84 |
| CORPUS UTERI | 2 | 1.46 | 1.37 | 2 | 1.46 | 1.37 |
| UTERUS,UNSPEC | 1 | 0.91 | 1.10 | 1 | 0.91 | 1.10 |
| OVARY | 0 | 1.40 | 0.0 | 0 | 1.40 | 0.0 |
| OTHER FEMALE GENITAL | 1 | 0.36 | 2.81 | 1 | 0.36 | 2.81 |
| PROSTATE | 0 | 0.0 | 0.0 | 0 | 0.0 | 0.0 |
| TESTIS | 0 | 0.0 | 0.0 | 0 | 0.0 | 0.0 |
| OTHER MALE GENITAL | 0 | 0.0 | 0.0 | 0 | 0.0 | 0.0 |
| KIDNEY AND URETER | 0 | 0.47 | 0.0 | 0 | 0.47 | 0.0 |
| BLADDER | 1 | 1.00 | 1.00 | 1 | 1.00 | 1.00 |
| MELANOMA OF SKIN | 1 | 0.24 | 4.26 | 1 | 0.24 | 4.26 |
| EYE | 0 | 0.06 | 0.0 | 0 | 0.06 | 0.0 |
| NERVOUS SYSTEM | 1 | 0.28 | 3.54 | 1 | 0.28 | 3.54 |
| THYROID | 0 | 0.24 | 0.0 | 0 | 0.24 | 0.0 |
| BONE | 0 | 0.09 | 0.0 | 0 | 0.09 | 0.0 |
| SOFT TISSUE | 1 | 0.19 | 5.38 | 1 | 0.19 | 5.38 |
| LYMPHOMAS & MYELOMA | 1 | 0.79 | 1.26 | 1 | 0.79 | 1.26 |
| LEUKEMIAS | 0 | 0.75 | 0.0 | 0 | 0.75 | 0.0 |
| OTHER SITES | 3 | 1.93 | 1.56 | 3 | 1.93 | 1.56 |
| TOTAL | 28 | 32.47 | 0.86 | 28 | 32.47 | 0.86 |

Table 80. Subsequent primary sites with excesses

FIRST PRIMARY SITE - OTHER AND UNSPECIFIED FEMALE GENITAL ORGANS

| SUBSEQUENT PRIMARY SITES | TOTAL | | | YEARS < 1 | | | YEARS 1-5 | | | YEARS > 5 | | |
|---|---|---|---|---|---|---|---|---|---|---|---|---|
| | NUMBER OF PERSONS= 852 PERSON-YRS OF OBSERVATION= 3946.0 | | | NUMBER OF PERSONS= 852 PERSON-YRS OF OBSERVATION= 706.5 | | | NUMBER OF PERSONS= 579 PERSON-YRS OF OBSERVATION= 1472.0 | | | NUMBER OF PERSONS= 257 PERSON-YRS OF OBSERVATION= 1767.5 | | |
| | OBS | EXP | OBS/EXP | OBS | EXP | OBS/EXP | OBS | EXP | OBS/EXP | OBS | EXP | OBS/EXP |
| ESOPHAGUS | 2 | 0.20 | 10.00* | 0 | 0.04 | 0.0 | 0 | 0.08 | 0.0 | 2 | 0.09 | 22.88** |

Table 81. Histologic confirmation of multiple primary malignancies

FIRST PRIMARY SITE - OTHER AND UNSPECIFIED FEMALE GENITAL ORGANS

| Subsequent primary site | Both tumors microscopically confirmed | | Only 1st tumor microscopically confirmed | | Only 2nd tumor microscopically confirmed | | Neither tumor microscopically confirmed | |
|---|---|---|---|---|---|---|---|---|
| | No. | % | No. | % | No. | % | No. | % |
| ESOPHAGUS | 1 | 50.0 | 1 | 50.0 | 0 | 0.0 | 0 | 0.0 |

Table 82. Subsequent multiple primary malignancies in patients with an index malignant tumor of the prostate

FIRST PRIMARY SITE - PROSTATE

| SUBSEQUENT PRIMARY SITES | TOTAL NUMBER OF PERSONS= 7249 PERSON-YRS OF OBSERVATION = 22930.1 OBS | EXP | OBS/EXP | MALES NUMBER OF PERSONS= 7249 PERSON-YRS OF OBSERVATION = 22930.1 OBS | EXP | OBS/EXP |
|---|---|---|---|---|---|---|
| LIP | 7 | 6.49 | 1.08 | 7 | 6.49 | 1.08 |
| TONGUE | 5 | 4.93 | 1.01 | 5 | 4.93 | 1.01 |
| SALIVARY GLAND | 3 | 1.22 | 2.46 | 3 | 1.22 | 2.46 |
| MOUTH | 7 | 6.51 | 1.07 | 7 | 6.51 | 1.07 |
| PHARYNX | 4 | 5.97 | 0.67 | 4 | 5.97 | 0.67 |
| ESOPHAGUS | 3 | 11.25 | 0.27** | 3 | 11.25 | 0.27** |
| STOMACH | 17 | 42.29 | 0.40** | 17 | 42.29 | 0.40** |
| SMALL INTESTINE | 3 | 1.25 | 2.40 | 3 | 1.25 | 2.40 |
| COLON | 36 | 50.10 | 0.72* | 36 | 50.10 | 0.72* |
| RECTUM | 29 | 30.70 | 0.94 | 29 | 30.70 | 0.94 |
| LIVER & BILIARY PASS | 2 | 9.23 | 0.22* | 2 | 9.23 | 0.22* |
| PANCREAS | 16 | 16.31 | 0.98 | 16 | 16.31 | 0.98 |
| NOSE AND SINUSES | 1 | 0.96 | 1.04 | 1 | 0.96 | 1.04 |
| LARYNX | 4 | 8.00 | 0.50 | 4 | 8.00 | 0.50 |
| LUNG AND BRONCHUS | 28 | 43.52 | 0.64* | 28 | 43.52 | 0.64* |
| OTHER RESP | 0 | 0.68 | 0.0 | 0 | 0.68 | 0.0 |
| BREAST | 1 | 0.95 | 1.05 | 1 | 0.95 | 1.05 |
| CERVIX UTERI | 0 | 0.0 | 0.0 | 0 | 0.0 | 0.0 |
| CORPUS UTERI | 0 | 0.0 | 0.0 | 0 | 0.0 | 0.0 |
| UTERUS,UNSPEC | 0 | 0.0 | 0.0 | 0 | 0.0 | 0.0 |
| OVARY | 0 | 0.0 | 0.0 | 0 | 0.0 | 0.0 |
| OTHER FEMALE GENITAL | 0 | 0.0 | 0.0 | 0 | 0.0 | 0.0 |
| PROSTATE | 0 | 93.98 | 0.0 | 0 | 93.98 | 0.0 |
| TESTIS | 1 | 0.56 | 1.79 | 1 | 0.56 | 1.79 |
| OTHER MALE GENITAL | 5 | 1.52 | 3.29* | 5 | 1.52 | 3.29* |
| KIDNEY AND URETER | 11 | 8.26 | 1.33 | 11 | 8.26 | 1.33 |
| BLADDER | 29 | 31.25 | 0.93 | 29 | 31.25 | 0.93 |
| MELANCMA OF SKIN | 5 | 2.07 | 2.41 | 5 | 2.07 | 2.41 |
| EYE | 0 | 0.67 | 0.0 | 0 | 0.67 | 0.0 |
| NERVOUS SYSTEM | 2 | 1.71 | 1.17 | 2 | 1.71 | 1.17 |
| THYROID | 0 | 0.97 | 0.0 | 0 | 0.97 | 0.0 |
| BONE | 0 | 0.98 | 0.0 | 0 | 0.98 | 0.0 |
| SOFT TISSUE | 0 | 2.43 | 0.0 | 0 | 2.43 | 0.0 |
| LYMPHOMAS & MYELOMA | 6 | 9.69 | 0.62 | 6 | 9.69 | 0.62 |
| LEUKEMIAS | 21 | 12.21 | 1.72* | 21 | 12.21 | 1.72* |
| OTHER SITES | 13 | 22.13 | 0.59 | 13 | 22.13 | 0.59 |
| TOTAL | 259 | 428.79 | 0.60** | 259 | 428.79 | 0.60** |

Table 83. Subsequent primary sites with excesses

FIRST PRIMARY SITE - PRCSTATE

| SUBSEQUENT PRIMARY SITES | TOTAL | | | YEARS < 1 | | | YEARS 1-5 | | | YEARS > 5 | | |
|---|---|---|---|---|---|---|---|---|---|---|---|---|
| | NUMBER OF PERSONS= 7249 PERSON-YRS OF OBSERVATION= 22930.1 | | | NUMBER OF PERSONS= 7249 PERSON-YRS OF OBSERVATION= 5974.4 | | | NUMBER OF PERSONS= 5129 PERSON-YRS OF OBSERVATICN= 11606.0 | | | NUMBER OF PERSONS= 1502 PERSON-YRS OF OBSERVATION= 5349.7 | | |
| | OBS | EXP | OBS/EXP | OBS | EXP | OBS/EXP | OBS | EXP | OBS/EXP | OBS | EXP | OBS/EXP |
| OTHER MALE GENITAL | 5 | 1.52 | 3.29* | 2 | 0.38 | 5.25 | 2 | 0.75 | 2.65 | 1 | 0.38 | 2.60 |
| LEUKEMIAS | 21 | 12.21 | 1.72* | 5 | 2.86 | 1.75 | 9 | 6.08 | 1.48 | 7 | 3.26 | 2.14 |

Table 84. Subsequent primary sites with deficiencies

FIRST PRIMARY SITE - PROSTATE

| SUBSEQUENT PRIMARY SITES | TOTAL | | | YEARS < 1 | | | YEARS 1-5 | | | YEARS > 5 | | |
|---|---|---|---|---|---|---|---|---|---|---|---|---|
| | NUMBER OF PERSONS= 7249 PERSON-YRS OF OBSERVATION= 22930.1 | | | NUMBER OF PERSONS= 7249 PERSON-YRS OF OBSERVATION= 5974.4 | | | NUMBER OF PERSONS= 5129 PERSON-YRS OF OBSERVATION= 11606.0 | | | NUMBER OF PERSONS= 1502 PERSON-YRS OF OBSEFVATICN= 5349.7 | | |
| | OBS | EXP | OBS/EXP | OBS | EXP | OBS/EXP | OBS | EXP | OBS/EXP | OBS | EXP | OBS/EXP |
| ESOPHAGUS | 3 | 11.25 | 0.27** | 2 | 2.80 | 0.71 | 0 | 5.69 | 0.0 | 1 | 2.76 | 0.36 |
| STOMACH | 17 | 42.29 | 0.40** | 8 | 10.39 | 0.77 | 6 | 21.04 | 0.29** | 3 | 10.86 | 0.28* |
| COLON | 36 | 50.10 | 0.72* | 8 | 11.81 | 0.68 | 15 | 24.87 | 0.60* | 13 | 13.42 | 0.97 |
| LIVER & BILIARY PASS | 2 | 9.23 | 0.22* | 0 | 2.24 | 0.0 | 1 | 4.59 | 0.22 | 1 | 2.40 | 0.42 |
| LUNG AND BRONCHUS | 28 | 43.52 | 0.64* | 3 | 10.58 | 0.28* | 14 | 22.13 | 0.63 | 11 | 10.81 | 1.02 |

Table 85. Histologic confirmation of multiple primary malignancies

FIRST PRIMARY SITE - PROSTATE

| Subsequent primary site | Both tumors micro-scopically confirmed | | Only 1st tumor micro-scopically confirmed | | Only 2nd tumor micro-scopically confirmed | | Neither tumor micro-scopically confirmed | |
|---|---|---|---|---|---|---|---|---|
| | No. | % | No. | % | No. | % | No. | % |
| OTHER MALE GENITAL | 5 | 100.0 | 0 | 0.0 | 0 | 0.0 | 0 | 0.0 |
| LEUKEMIAS | 15 | 71.4 | 1 | 4.8 | 3 | 14.3 | 2 | 9.5 |

Table 86. Subsequent multiple primary malignancies in patients with an index malignant tumor of the testis

FIRST PRIMARY SITE - TESTIS

| | TOTAL | | | MALES | | |
|---|---|---|---|---|---|---|
| | NUMBER OF PERSONS= 636 PERSON-YRS OF OBSERVATION = 3594.0 | | | NUMBER OF PERSONS= 636 PERSON-YRS OF OBSERVATION = 3594.0 | | |
| SUBSEQUENT PRIMARY SITES | OBS | EXP | OBS/EXP | OBS | EXP | OBS/EXP |
| LIP | 1 | 0.20 | 5.10 | 1 | 0.20 | 5.10 |
| TONGUE | 0 | 0.18 | 0.0 | 0 | 0.18 | 0.0 |
| SALIVARY GLAND | 0 | 0.05 | 0.0 | 0 | 0.05 | 0.0 |
| MOUTH | 0 | 0.20 | 0.0 | 0 | 0.20 | 0.0 |
| PHARYNX | 1 | 0.23 | 4.26 | 1 | 0.23 | 4.26 |
| ESOPHAGUS | 0 | 0.34 | 0.0 | 0 | 0.34 | 0.0 |
| STOMACH | 0 | 1.01 | 0.0 | 0 | 1.01 | 0.0 |
| SMALL INTESTINE | 0 | 0.05 | 0.0 | 0 | 0.05 | 0.0 |
| COLON | 4 | 1.22 | 3.28 | 4 | 1.22 | 3.28 |
| RECTUM | 3 | 0.86 | 3.50 | 3 | 0.86 | 3.50 |
| LIVER & BILIARY PASS | 1 | 0.22 | 4.50 | 1 | 0.22 | 4.50 |
| PANCREAS | 1 | 0.41 | 2.44 | 1 | 0.41 | 2.44 |
| NOSE AND SINUSES | 0 | 0.03 | 0.0 | 0 | 0.03 | 0.0 |
| LARYNX | 0 | 0.34 | 0.0 | 0 | 0.34 | 0.0 |
| LUNG AND BRONCHUS | 4 | 1.94 | 2.06 | 4 | 1.94 | 2.06 |
| OTHER RESP | 0 | 0.04 | 0.0 | 0 | 0.04 | 0.0 |
| BREAST | 0 | 0.03 | 0.0 | 0 | 0.03 | 0.0 |
| CERVIX UTERI | 0 | 0.0 | 0.0 | 0 | 0.0 | 0.0 |
| CORPUS UTERI | 0 | 0.0 | 0.0 | 0 | 0.0 | 0.0 |
| UTERUS,UNSPEC | 0 | 0.0 | 0.0 | 0 | 0.0 | 0.0 |
| OVARY | 0 | 0.0 | 0.0 | 0 | 0.0 | 0.0 |
| OTHER FEMALE GENITAL | 0 | 0.0 | 0.0 | 0 | 0.0 | 0.0 |
| PROSTATE | 3 | 1.22 | 2.47 | 3 | 1.22 | 2.47 |
| TESTIS | 1 | 0.13 | 7.68 | 1 | 0.13 | 7.68 |
| OTHER MALE GENITAL | 0 | 0.05 | 0.0 | 0 | 0.05 | 0.0 |
| KIDNEY AND URETER | 1 | 0.32 | 3.12 | 1 | 0.32 | 3.12 |
| BLADDER | 1 | 0.81 | 1.23 | 1 | 0.81 | 1.23 |
| MELANOMA OF SKIN | 0 | 0.14 | 0.0 | 0 | 0.14 | 0.0 |
| EYE | 0 | 0.03 | 0.0 | 0 | 0.03 | 0.0 |
| NERVOUS SYSTEM | 0 | 0.25 | 0.0 | 0 | 0.25 | 0.0 |
| THYROID | 0 | 0.05 | 0.0 | 0 | 0.05 | 0.0 |
| BONE | 0 | 0.04 | 0.0 | 0 | 0.04 | 0.0 |
| SOFT TISSUE | 1 | 0.11 | 8.73 | 1 | 0.11 | 8.73 |
| LYMPHOMAS & MYELOMA | 1 | 0.49 | 2.04 | 1 | 0.49 | 2.04 |
| LEUKEMIAS | 3 | 0.40 | 7.58* | 3 | 0.40 | 7.58* |
| OTHER SITES | 1 | 0.65 | 1.54 | 1 | 0.65 | 1.54 |
| TOTAL | 27 | 12.03 | 2.25** | 27 | 12.03 | 2.25** |

Table 87. Subsequent primary sites with excesses

FIRST PRIMARY SITE - TESTIS

| SUBSEQUENT PRIMARY SITES | TOTAL<br>NUMBER OF PERSONS= 636<br>PERSON-YRS OF OBSERVATION= 3594.0 | | | YEARS < 1<br>NUMBER OF PERSONS= 636<br>PERSON-YRS OF OBSERVATION= 543.6 | | | YEARS 1-5<br>NUMBER OF PERSONS= 461<br>PERSON-YRS OF OBSERVATICN= 1264.2 | | | YEARS > 5<br>NUMBER OF PERSONS= 238<br>PERSCN-YRS CF OBSERVATION= 1786.2 | | |
|---|---|---|---|---|---|---|---|---|---|---|---|---|
| | OBS | EXP | OBS/EXP | OBS | EXP | OBS/EXP | OBS | EXP | OBS/EXP | OPS | EXP | OBS/EXP |
| PHARYNX | 1 | 0.23 | 4.26 | 1 | 0.02 | 49.95* | 0 | 0.06 | 0.0 | 0 | 0.16 | 0.0 |
| COLON | 4 | 1.22 | 3.28 | 2 | 0.10 | 19.51** | 0 | 0.27 | 0.0 | 2 | C.84 | 2.37 |
| LIVER & BILIARY PASS | 1 | 0.22 | 4.50 | 1 | 0.02 | 51.31* | 0 | 0.05 | 0.C | 0 | 0.15 | 0.0 |
| LEUKEMIAS | 3 | 0.40 | 7.58* | 0 | 0.04 | 0.0 | 0 | 0.10 | 0.0 | 3 | 0.26 | 11.59** |

Table 88. Histologic confirmation of multiple primary malignancies

FIRST PRIMARY SITE - TESTIS

| Subsequent primary site | Both tumors microscopically confirmed | | Only 1st tumor microscopically confirmed | | Only 2nd tumor microscopically confirmed | | Neither tumor microscopically confirmed | |
|---|---|---|---|---|---|---|---|---|
| | No. | % | No. | % | No. | % | No. | % |
| PHARYNX | 1 | 100.0 | 0 | 0.0 | 0 | 0.0 | 0 | 0.0 |
| COLON | 3 | 75.0 | 1 | 25.0 | 0 | 0.0 | 0 | 0.0 |
| LIVER & BILIARY PASS | 0 | 0.0 | 1 | 100.0 | 0 | 0.0 | 0 | 0.0 |
| LEUKEMIAS | 3 | 100.0 | 0 | 0.0 | 0 | 0.0 | 0 | 0.0 |

Table 89. Subsequent multiple primary malignancies in patients with an index malignant tumor of other and unspecified male genital organs

FIRST PRIMARY SITE - OTHER AND UNSPECIFIED MALE GENITAL ORGANS

| | TOTAL | | | MALES | | |
|---|---|---|---|---|---|---|
| | NUMBER OF PERSONS= 343<br>PERSON-YRS OF<br>OBSERVATION = 1790.8 | | | NUMBER OF PERSONS= 343<br>PERSON-YRS OF<br>OBSERVATION = 1790.8 | | |
| SUBSEQUENT PRIMARY SITES | OBS | EXP | OBS/EXP | OBS | EXP | OBS/EXP |
| LIP | 0 | 0.37 | 0.0 | 0 | 0.37 | 0.0 |
| TONGUE | 1 | 0.28 | 3.62 | 1 | 0.28 | 3.62 |
| SALIVARY GLAND | 0 | 0.07 | 0.0 | 0 | 0.07 | 0.0 |
| MOUTH | 0 | 0.36 | 0.0 | 0 | 0.36 | 0.0 |
| PHARYNX | 0 | 0.35 | 0.0 | 0 | 0.35 | 0.0 |
| ESOPHAGUS | 0 | 0.63 | 0.0 | 0 | 0.63 | 0.0 |
| STOMACH | 1 | 2.21 | 0.45 | 1 | 2.21 | 0.45 |
| SMALL INTESTINE | 0 | 0.07 | 0.0 | 0 | 0.07 | 0.0 |
| COLON | 4 | 2.51 | 1.59 | 4 | 2.51 | 1.59 |
| RECTUM | 0 | 1.63 | 0.0 | 0 | 1.63 | 0.0 |
| LIVER & BILIARY PASS | 0 | 0.48 | 0.0 | 0 | 0.48 | 0.0 |
| PANCREAS | 0 | 0.83 | 0.0 | 0 | 0.83 | 0.0 |
| NOSE AND SINUSES | 0 | 0.05 | 0.0 | 0 | 0.05 | 0.0 |
| LARYNX | 1 | 0.49 | 2.03 | 1 | 0.49 | 2.03 |
| LUNG AND BRONCHUS | 6 | 2.71 | 2.22 | 6 | 2.71 | 2.22 |
| OTHER RESP | 0 | 0.04 | 0.0 | 0 | 0.04 | 0.0 |
| BREAST | 0 | 0.05 | 0.0 | 0 | 0.05 | 0.0 |
| CERVIX UTERI | 0 | 0.0 | 0.0 | 0 | 0.0 | 0.0 |
| CORPUS UTERI | 0 | 0.0 | 0.0 | 0 | 0.0 | 0.0 |
| UTERUS,UNSPEC | 0 | 0.0 | 0.0 | 0 | 0.0 | 0.0 |
| OVARY | 0 | 0.0 | 0.0 | 0 | 0.0 | 0.0 |
| OTHER FEMALE GENITAL | 0 | 0.0 | 0.0 | 0 | 0.0 | 0.0 |
| PROSTATE | 10 | 4.09 | 2.44* | 10 | 4.09 | 2.44* |
| TESTIS | 0 | 0.04 | 0.0 | 0 | 0.04 | 0.0 |
| OTHER MALE GENITAL | 0 | 0.09 | 0.0 | 0 | 0.09 | 0.0 |
| KIDNEY AND URETER | 0 | 0.46 | 0.0 | 0 | 0.46 | 0.0 |
| BLADDER | 2 | 1.59 | 1.26 | 2 | 1.59 | 1.26 |
| MELANOMA OF SKIN | 0 | 0.12 | 0.0 | 0 | 0.12 | 0.0 |
| EYE | 0 | 0.04 | 0.0 | 0 | 0.04 | 0.0 |
| NERVOUS SYSTEM | 0 | 0.17 | 0.0 | 0 | 0.17 | 0.0 |
| THYROID | 1 | 0.06 | 17.49 | 1 | 0.06 | 17.49 |
| BONE | 0 | 0.06 | 0.0 | 0 | 0.06 | 0.0 |
| SOFT TISSUE | 0 | 0.13 | 0.0 | 0 | 0.13 | 0.0 |
| LYMPHOMAS & MYELOMA | 0 | 0.55 | 0.0 | 0 | 0.55 | 0.0 |
| LEUKEMIAS | 0 | 0.63 | 0.0 | 0 | 0.63 | 0.0 |
| OTHER SITES | 1 | 1.16 | 0.86 | 1 | 1.16 | 0.86 |
| TOTAL | 27 | 22.32 | 1.21 | 27 | 22.32 | 1.21 |

Table 90. Subsequent primary sites with excesses

FIRST PRIMARY SITE - OTHER AND UNSPECIFIED MALE GENITAL ORGANS

| SUBSEQUENT PRIMARY SITES | TOTAL<br>NUMBER OF PERSONS= 343<br>PERSON-YRS OF OBSERVATION= 1790.8 | | | YEARS < 1<br>NUMBER OF PERSONS= 343<br>PERSON-YRS OF OBSERVATION= 305.6 | | | YEARS 1-5<br>NUMBER OF PERSONS= 270<br>PERSON-YRS OF OBSERVATION= 755.2 | | | YEARS > 5<br>NUMBER OF PERSONS= 137<br>PERSON-YRS OF OBSERVATION= 730.1 | | |
|---|---|---|---|---|---|---|---|---|---|---|---|---|
| | OBS | EXP | OBS/EXP | OBS | EXP | OBS/EXP | OBS | EXP | OBS/EXP | OBS | EXP | OBS/EXP |
| PROSTATE | 10 | 4.09 | 2.44* | 1 | 0.61 | 1.64 | 5 | 1.64 | 3.05 | 4 | 1.84 | 2.17 |

Table 91. Histologic confirmation of multiple primary malignancies

FIRST PRIMARY SITE - OTHER AND UNSPECIFIED MALE GENITAL ORGANS

| Subsequent primary site | Both tumors microscopically confirmed | | Only 1st tumor microscopically confirmed | | Only 2nd tumor microscopically confirmed | | Neither tumor microscopically confirmed | |
|---|---|---|---|---|---|---|---|---|
| | No. | % | No. | % | No. | % | No. | % |
| PROSTATE | 7 | 70.0 | 3 | 30.0 | 0 | 0.0 | 0 | 0.0 |

Table 92. Summary of site-group pairs with an excess of observed-over-expected subsequent primary malignancies: index tumors of the breast and reproductive organs

I. Possibly artifact

| | | |
|---|---|---|
| Breast | ⟶ | Tongue |
| Breast | ⟶ | Bladder |
| Cervix | ⟶ | Other/unspecified sites |
| Other/unspecified female genital organs | ⟶ | Esophagus |
| Testis | ⟷ | Pharynx |
| Testis | ⟶ | Colon |
| Testis | ⟶ | Liver/biliary passages |

II. Possibly real

A. In organs within the same system

1. Same or paired organs

| | | |
|---|---|---|
| Breast | ⟷ | Breast |

2. Others

| | | |
|---|---|---|
| Corpus uteri | ⟷ | Ovary |
| Cervix uteri | ⟶ | Other/unspecified female genital organs |
| Corpus uteri | ⟶ | Other/unspecified female genital organs |
| Prostate | ⟷ | Other/unspecified male genital organs |

B. In organs related structurally or functionally

| | | |
|---|---|---|
| Breast | ⟷ | Corpus uteri |
| Breast | ⟶ | Ovary |

C. In organs apparently unrelated structurally or functionally

| | | |
|---|---|---|
| Corpus uteri | ⟷ | Colon |
| Ovary | ⟷ | Colon |
| Breast | ⟶ | Colon |
| Breast | ⟶ | Soft tissue |
| Cervix uteri | ⟶ | Rectum |
| Corpus uteri | ⟶ | Rectum |
| Corpus uteri | ⟶ | Kidney/ureter |
| Cervix uteri | ⟶ | Pharynx |
| Cervix uteri | ⟶ | Lung/bronchus |
| Cervix uteri | ⟶ | Bladder |
| Prostate | ⟷ | Leukemia |
| Testis | ⟶ | Leukemia |
| Breast | ⟶ | Eye |

Table 93. Summary of site-group pairs with a deficiency of observed-over-expected subsequent primary malignancies: index tumors of the breast and reproductive organs

| | |
|---|---|
| Breast → | Pancreas |
| Breast → | Nervous system |
| Breast → | Other/unspecified sites |
| Cervix uteri → | Liver/biliary passages |
| Corpus uteri → | Stomach |
| Corpus uteri → | Cervix uteri |
| Prostate → | Esophagus |
| Prostate → | Stomach |
| Prostate → | Colon |
| Prostate → | Liver/biliary passages |
| Prostate → | Lung/bronchus |

Table 94. Common metastatic sites for primary malignant tumors of the breast and reproductive organs (HOLLAND and FREI, 1973; WILLIS, 1973; RUBIN, 1974)

| Anatomic location of the primary malignant tumor | Common metastatic sites |
|---|---|
| Breast | Axillary lymph nodes; other breast; lung; liver; bone; thyroid; eye |
| Cervix uteri | External iliac, hypogastric, periaortic, and pelvic lymph nodes; cardinal ligaments; lung; bone; bladder; rectum |
| Corpus uteri | Myometrium; ovary; pelvic and periaortic lymph nodes; cervix; vagina; bladder; rectum |
| Ovary | Periaortic nodes; fallopian tube; corpus uteri; within abdomen (omentum, small intestine, and mesentery); opposite ovary |
| Other female genital organs | Hypogastric, iliac, inguinal and femoral lymph nodes; cervix; vagina; vulva; lateral pelvic walls; urethra; bladder; rectum; anus; bone |
| Prostate | Obturator, hypogastric, periaortic, and pelvic lymph nodes; ureter; bone; vertebral column; thoracic spine; skull |
| Testis and penis | Inguinal, external iliac, common iliac, femoral, and periaortic lymph nodes; lung; liver |

# Chapter 10

# Index Tumors of the Urinary System

Population Studied. 5,849 males and 2,419 females with cancer of the urinary system were followed for the subsequent development of independent primary malignant neoplasms; 468 such subsequent neoplasms were discovered. The cohort of patients with cancer of the urinary system contributed 32,669 person-years of observation.

Results. Detailed tabulations by site are presented in Tables 95-101. The reader is referred to Chapter 5 for a general explanation of the items in these tables.

Summary of Findings. Site-group pairs with a statistically significant excess of observed-over-expected subsequent primary cancers are categorized in Table 102 on the basis of possible relationships between the anatomic sites containing these cancers. In addition, possible artifactual relationships, based on a small number of cases and with no confirmation from other published reports, are emphasized.

Discussion. Table 103 presents the common metastatic sites for cancers arising within the urinary system. These data, used in conjunction with the site-specific tabulations of the percentage of multiple primary malignancies with histologic confirmation, are useful in distinguishing real from artifactual associations.

The site-group pairs listed in category I are based on very few cases, and are not supported by other published studies. All patients in this category had microscopic confirmation of both the first and subsequent primary malignancies, so it is doubtful that metastatic disease would have been mistaken for a new, independent primary cancer. Nevertheless, these associations are thought to be spurious.

Multiple primary cancers involving the same or different organs within the urinary system are a well-recognized phenomenon (MOERTEL, 1966). The site-group pairs listed in category IIA represent bidirectional associations and suggest that the same oncogenic factor is operating in the development of both cancers.

The excess risk of prostatic cancer in patients with an index malignancy of the urinary tract may be artifactual. It may represent the discovery of clinically silent prostatic malignancies during the autopsy examination. Moreover, it may be that patients dying with cancer of the urinary system come to autopsy more frequently than the general population of deaths. The excess risk of testicular cancer following a malignancy of the kidney or ureter is represented by only one patient in whom both tumors were histologically verified. Although the associations in category IIB may be spurious, the close functional and anatomic relationships of the involved organs suggest that there may be an underlying biologic mechanism for this relationship.

Site-group pairs listed in category IIC may be linked through a common etiologic agent: cigarette smoking. Smoking is known to increase the risk for cancer of the bladder (LILIENFELD et al., 1956; HAMMOND, 1966; LEVIN et al., 1974; HAMMOND, 1975), lung and bronchus (HAMMOND, 1966; LEVIN et al., 1974; HAMMOND, 1975), and oral cavity (LEVIN et al., 1974; HAMMOND, 1975). Since lung and bladder cancer are strongly correlated with smoking, one might expect to find a relationship between these tumors. In the present tabulations, the associations are unidirectional; i.e., patients with bladder cancer are at increased risk for cancer of the tongue or lung/bronchus, and not vice versa. The reason for this may be that patients with lung cancer do not live long enough to develop bladder cancer. Another explanation may be that following exposure to the carcinogenic agent, the latent period for developing apparent bladder cancer may be shorter than for developing clinically apparent cancer of the tongue or lung/bronchus.

Only one statistically significant deficiency of observed-over-expected subsequent primary cancers was found, namely a decreased risk of bladder cancer subsequent to an initial bladder cancer. Multicentric bladder malignancies discovered at the same time are described in Chapter 3. The deficit found in the Connecticut data is probably artifactual, and may represent operative removal of the urinary bladder in whole or in part as treatment for the initial neoplasm. The patient would be at no further risk for developing cancer at that site if the organ were totally removed. The phenomenon of multiple primary bladder tumors (not shown in the present analysis of non-simultaneously diagnosed multiple primaries) is substantially documented in the literature (MOERTEL, 1966).

Table 95. Subsequent multiple primary malignancies in patients with an index malignant tumor of the kidney and ureter

FIRST PRIMARY SITE - KIDNEY AND URETER

| | TOTAL | | | MALES | | | FEMALES | | |
|---|---|---|---|---|---|---|---|---|---|
| | NUMBER OF PERSONS= 2272 PERSON-YRS OF OBSERVATION = 6893.2 | | | NUMBER OF PERSONS= 1431 PERSON-YRS OF OBSERVATION = 4211.2 | | | NUMBER OF PERSONS= 841 PERSON-YRS OF OBSERVATION = 2681.9 | | |
| SUBSEQUENT PRIMARY SITES | OBS | EXP | OBS/EXP | OBS | EXP | OBS/EXP | OBS | EXP | OBS/EXP |
| LIP | 3 | 0.65 | 4.64 | 3 | 0.62 | 4.85 | 0 | 0.03 | 0.0 |
| TONGUE | 0 | 0.59 | 0.0 | 0 | 0.54 | 0.0 | 0 | 0.06 | 0.0 |
| SALIVARY GLAND | 0 | 0.18 | 0.0 | 0 | 0.12 | 0.0 | 0 | 0.06 | 0.0 |
| MOUTH | 1 | 0.74 | 1.34 | 1 | 0.65 | 1.53 | 0 | 0.09 | 0.0 |
| PHARYNX | 1 | 0.76 | 1.31 | 1 | 0.68 | 1.47 | 0 | 0.08 | 0.0 |
| ESOPHAGUS | 0 | 1.30 | 0.0 | 0 | 1.19 | 0.0 | 0 | 0.12 | 0.0 |
| STOMACH | 3 | 5.17 | 0.58 | 3 | 3.85 | 0.78 | 0 | 1.32 | 0.0 |
| SMALL INTESTINE | 0 | 0.22 | 0.0 | 0 | 0.14 | 0.0 | 0 | 0.08 | 0.0 |
| COLON | 8 | 7.71 | 1.04 | 4 | 4.69 | 0.85 | 4 | 3.01 | 1.33 |
| RECTUM | 3 | 4.31 | 0.70 | 2 | 3.02 | 0.66 | 1 | 1.29 | 0.78 |
| LIVER & BILIARY PASS | 1 | 1.48 | 0.67 | 0 | 0.86 | 0.0 | 1 | 0.63 | 1.59 |
| PANCREAS | 1 | 2.24 | 0.45 | 1 | 1.57 | 0.64 | 0 | 0.67 | 0.0 |
| NOSE AND SINUSES | 0 | 0.13 | 0.0 | 0 | 0.09 | 0.0 | 0 | 0.04 | 0.0 |
| LARYNX | 0 | 1.05 | 0.0 | 0 | 1.01 | 0.0 | 0 | 0.04 | 0.0 |
| LUNG AND BRONCHUS | 7 | 6.41 | 1.09 | 6 | 5.86 | 1.02 | 1 | 0.54 | 1.84 |
| OTHER RESP | 0 | 0.10 | 0.0 | 0 | 0.09 | 0.0 | 0 | 0.02 | 0.0 |
| BREAST | 6 | 4.94 | 1.21 | 0 | 0.11 | 0.0 | 6 | 4.84 | 1.24 |
| CERVIX UTERI | 1 | 1.18 | 0.85 | 0 | 0.0 | 0.0 | 1 | 1.18 | 0.85 |
| CORPUS UTERI | 0 | 1.10 | 0.0 | 0 | 0.0 | 0.0 | 0 | 1.10 | 0.0 |
| UTERUS,UNSPEC | 1 | 0.55 | 1.81 | 0 | 0.0 | 0.0 | 1 | 0.55 | 1.81 |
| OVARY | 1 | 0.98 | 1.02 | 0 | 0.0 | 0.0 | 1 | 0.98 | 1.02 |
| OTHER FEMALE GENITAL | 0 | 0.22 | 0.0 | 0 | 0.0 | 0.0 | 0 | 0.22 | 0.0 |
| PROSTATE | 17 | 6.96 | 2.44** | 17 | 6.96 | 2.44** | 0 | 0.0 | 0.0 |
| TESTIS | 1 | 0.09 | 10.78 | 1 | 0.09 | 10.78 | 0 | 0.0 | 0.0 |
| OTHER MALE GENITAL | 0 | 0.14 | 0.0 | 0 | 0.14 | 0.0 | 0 | 0.0 | 0.0 |
| KIDNEY AND URETER | 3 | 1.29 | 2.32 | 1 | 0.97 | 1.03 | 2 | 0.32 | 6.20 |
| BLADDER | 29 | 3.61 | 8.04** | 17 | 3.01 | 5.65** | 12 | 0.60 | 20.07** |
| MELANOMA OF SKIN | 1 | 0.41 | 2.46 | 0 | 0.25 | 0.0 | 1 | 0.16 | 6.22 |
| EYE | 0 | 0.12 | 0.0 | 0 | 0.08 | 0.0 | 0 | 0.04 | 0.0 |
| NERVOUS SYSTEM | 1 | 0.60 | 1.68 | 0 | 0.39 | 0.0 | 1 | 0.20 | 4.88 |
| THYROID | 0 | 0.27 | 0.0 | 0 | 0.12 | 0.0 | 0 | 0.15 | 0.0 |
| BONE | 1 | 0.16 | 6.21 | 1 | 0.10 | 9.59 | 0 | 0.06 | 0.0 |
| SOFT TISSUE | 2 | 0.42 | 4.81 | 2 | 0.28 | 7.07 | 0 | 0.13 | 0.0 |
| LYMPHOMAS & MYELOMA | 1 | 1.73 | 0.58 | 1 | 1.16 | 0.87 | 0 | 0.57 | 0.0 |
| LEUKEMIAS | 1 | 1.79 | 0.56 | 1 | 1.27 | 0.79 | 0 | 0.52 | 0.0 |
| OTHER SITES | 6 | 3.48 | 1.72 | 5 | 2.26 | 2.21 | 1 | 1.22 | 0.82 |
| TOTAL | 100 | 63.07 | 1.59** | 67 | 42.18 | 1.59** | 33 | 20.89 | 1.58** |

Table 96. Subsequent primary sites with excesses

FIRST PRIMARY SITE - KIDNEY AND UFETER

| SUBSEQUENT PRIMARY SITES | TOTAL | | | YEARS < 1 | | | YEARS 1-5 | | | YEARS > 5 | | |
|---|---|---|---|---|---|---|---|---|---|---|---|---|
| | NUMBER OF PERSONS= 2272 PERSON-YRS OF OBSERVATION= 6893.2 | | | NUMBER OF PERSONS= 2272 PERSON-YRS OF OBSERVATION= 1616.2 | | | NUMBER OF PERSONS= 1224 PERSON-YRS OF OBSERVATICN= 2923.1 | | | NUMBER OF PERSONS= 460 PERSON-YRS OF OBSERVATION= 2353.9 | | |
| | OBS | EXP | OBS/EXP | OBS | EXP | OBS/EXP | OBS | EXP | OBS/EXP | OBS | EXP | OBS/EXP |
| PROSTATE | 17 | 6.96 | 2.44** | 5 | 1.46 | 3.42* | 7 | 2.94 | 2.38 | 5 | 2.56 | 1.95 |
| TESTIS | 1 | 0.09 | 10.78 | 1 | 0.02 | 42.96* | 0 | 0.04 | 0.0 | 0 | 0.03 | 0.0 |
| KIDNEY AND URETER | 3 | 1.29 | 2.32 | 3 | 0.29 | 10.40** | 0 | 0.54 | 0.0 | 0 | 0.47 | 0.0 |
| BLADDER | 29 | 3.61 | 8.04** | 8 | 0.79 | 10.15** | 17 | 1.50 | 11.33** | 4 | 1.32 | 3.04 |
| SOFT TISSUE | 2 | 0.42 | 4.81 | 2 | 0.09 | 22.56** | 0 | 0.17 | 0.0 | 0 | 0.16 | 0.0 |

Table 97. Histologic confirmation of multiple primary malignancies

FIRST PRIMARY SITE - KIDNEY AND URETER

| Subsequent primary site | Both tumors microscopically confirmed | | Only 1st tumor microscopically confirmed | | Only 2nd tumor microscopically confirmed | | Neither tumor microscopically confirmed | |
|---|---|---|---|---|---|---|---|---|
| | No. | % | No. | % | No. | % | No. | % |
| PROSTATE | 14 | 82.4 | 3 | 17.6 | 0 | 0.0 | 0 | 0.0 |
| TESTIS | 1 | 100.0 | 0 | 0.0 | 0 | 0.0 | 0 | 0.0 |
| KIDNEY AND URETER | 3 | 100.0 | 0 | 0.0 | 0 | 0.0 | 0 | 0.0 |
| BLADDER | 25 | 86.2 | 2 | 6.9 | 1 | 3.4 | 1 | 3.4 |
| SOFT TISSUE | 2 | 100.0 | 0 | 0.0 | 0 | 0.0 | 0 | 0.0 |

Table 98. Subsequent multiple primary malignancies in patients with an index malignant tumor of the bladder

FIRST PRIMARY SITE - BLADDER

| SUBSEQUENT PRIMARY SITES | TOTAL | | | MALES | | | FEMALES | | |
|---|---|---|---|---|---|---|---|---|---|
| | NUMBER OF PERSONS= 5996 PERSON-YRS OF OBSERVATION = 25775.7 | | | NUMBER OF PERSONS= 4418 PERSON-YRS OF OBSERVATION = 18704.6 | | | NUMBER OF PERSONS= 1578 PERSON-YRS OF OBSERVATION = 7071.2 | | |
| | OBS | EXP | OBS/EXP | OBS | EXP | OBS/EXP | OBS | EXP | OBS/EXP |
| LIP | 2 | 3.67 | 0.55 | 2 | 3.57 | 0.56 | 0 | 0.10 | 0.0 |
| TONGUE | 9 | 3.11 | 2.89** | 9 | 2.93 | 3.07** | 0 | 0.18 | 0.0 |
| SALIVARY GLAND | 1 | 0.89 | 1.13 | 1 | 0.69 | 1.45 | 0 | 0.20 | 0.0 |
| MOUTH | 4 | 4.03 | 0.99 | 4 | 3.70 | 1.08 | 0 | 0.33 | 0.0 |
| PHARYNX | 3 | 3.96 | 0.76 | 3 | 3.72 | 0.81 | 0 | 0.24 | 0.0 |
| ESOPHAGUS | 4 | 7.11 | 0.56 | 3 | 6.70 | 0.45 | 1 | 0.41 | 2.42 |
| STOMACH | 21 | 27.39 | 0.77 | 17 | 22.48 | 0.76 | 4 | 4.91 | 0.81 |
| SMALL INTESTINE | 0 | 1.04 | 0.0 | 0 | 0.78 | 0.0 | 0 | 0.27 | 0.0 |
| COLON | 41 | 37.73 | 1.09 | 32 | 27.34 | 1.17 | 9 | 10.39 | 0.87 |
| RECTUM | 24 | 21.54 | 1.11 | 21 | 17.30 | 1.21 | 3 | 4.25 | 0.71 |
| LIVER & BILIARY PASS | 6 | 7.27 | 0.83 | 5 | 5.02 | 1.00 | 1 | 2.25 | 0.44 |
| PANCREAS | 12 | 11.30 | 1.06 | 11 | 9.02 | 1.22 | 1 | 2.28 | 0.44 |
| NOSE AND SINUSES | 1 | 0.64 | 1.57 | 0 | 0.53 | 0.0 | 1 | 0.11 | 8.97 |
| LARYNX | 10 | 5.44 | 1.84 | 10 | 5.33 | 1.88 | 0 | 0.12 | 0.0 |
| LUNG AND BRONCHUS | 44 | 32.73 | 1.34* | 41 | 30.97 | 1.32 | 3 | 1.76 | 1.71 |
| OTHER RESP | 1 | 0.51 | 1.95 | 1 | 0.46 | 2.16 | 0 | 0.05 | 0.0 |
| BREAST | 17 | 15.76 | 1.08 | 0 | 0.58 | 0.0 | 17 | 15.19 | 1.12 |
| CERVIX UTERI | 4 | 3.15 | 1.27 | 0 | 0.0 | 0.0 | 4 | 3.15 | 1.27 |
| CORPUS UTERI | 4 | 3.06 | 1.31 | 0 | 0.0 | 0.0 | 4 | 3.06 | 1.31 |
| UTERUS,UNSPEC | 2 | 1.80 | 1.11 | 0 | 0.0 | 0.0 | 2 | 1.80 | 1.11 |
| OVARY | 3 | 2.79 | 1.07 | 0 | 0.0 | 0.0 | 3 | 2.79 | 1.07 |
| OTHER FEMALE GENITAL | 0 | 0.76 | 0.0 | 0 | 0.0 | 0.0 | 0 | 0.76 | 0.0 |
| PROSTATE | 88 | 44.42 | 1.98** | 88 | 44.42 | 1.98** | 0 | 0.0 | 0.0 |
| TESTIS | 1 | 0.45 | 2.21 | 1 | 0.45 | 2.21 | 0 | 0.0 | 0.0 |
| OTHER MALE GENITAL | 0 | 0.85 | 0.0 | 0 | 0.85 | 0.0 | 0 | 0.0 | 0.0 |
| KIDNEY AND URETER | 19 | 6.23 | 3.05** | 15 | 5.21 | 2.88** | 4 | 1.02 | 3.94* |
| BLADDER | 1 | 19.62 | 0.05** | 1 | 17.44 | 0.06** | 0 | 2.18 | 0.0 |
| MELANOMA OF SKIN | 1 | 1.78 | 0.56 | 1 | 1.31 | 0.77 | 0 | 0.48 | 0.0 |
| EYE | 0 | 0.54 | 0.0 | 0 | 0.41 | 0.0 | 0 | 0.14 | 0.0 |
| NERVOUS SYSTEM | 2 | 2.28 | 0.88 | 1 | 1.74 | 0.57 | 1 | 0.54 | 1.85 |
| THYROID | 2 | 1.13 | 1.77 | 2 | 0.63 | 3.15 | 0 | 0.50 | 0.0 |
| BONE | 2 | 0.74 | 2.70 | 1 | 0.56 | 1.79 | 1 | 0.18 | 5.47 |
| SOFT TISSUE | 1 | 1.92 | 0.52 | 0 | 1.53 | 0.0 | 1 | 0.39 | 2.56 |
| LYMPHOMAS & MYELOMA | 10 | 7.91 | 1.26 | 10 | 6.21 | 1.61 | 0 | 1.70 | 0.0 |
| LEUKEMIAS | 8 | 8.71 | 0.92 | 7 | 7.08 | 0.99 | 1 | 1.63 | 0.61 |
| OTHER SITES | 20 | 17.17 | 1.16 | 15 | 12.94 | 1.16 | 5 | 4.23 | 1.18 |
| TOTAL | 368 | 309.43 | 1.19** | 302 | 241.88 | 1.25** | 66 | 67.56 | 0.98 |

Table 99. Subsequent primary sites with excesses

FIRST PRIMARY SITE - BLADDER

| SUBSEQUENT PRIMARY SITES | TOTAL<br>NUMBER OF PERSONS= 5996<br>PERSON-YRS OF OBSERVATION= 25775.7 | | | YEARS < 1<br>NUMBER OF PERSONS= 5996<br>PERSON-YRS OF OBSERVATION= 4823.7 | | | YEARS 1-5<br>NUMBER OF PERSONS= 4017<br>PERSON-YRS OF OBSERVATION= 10737.2 | | | YEARS > 5<br>NUMBER OF PERSONS= 1861<br>PERSON-YRS OF OBSERVATION= 10214.8 | | |
|---|---|---|---|---|---|---|---|---|---|---|---|---|
| | OBS | EXP | OBS/EXP | OBS | EXP | OBS/EXP | OBS | EXP | OBS/EXP | OBS | EXP | OBS/EXP |
| TONGUE | 9 | 3.11 | 2.89** | 1 | 0.58 | 1.73 | 3 | 1.27 | 2.36 | 5 | 1.26 | 3.96* |
| LUNG AND BRONCHUS | 44 | 32.73 | 1.34* | 3 | 5.71 | 0.52 | 22 | 13.31 | 1.65* | 19 | 13.71 | 1.39 |
| CORPUS UTERI | 4 | 3.06 | 1.31 | 3 | 0.51 | 5.87* | 0 | 1.18 | 0.0 | 1 | 1.36 | 0.73 |
| PROSTATE | 88 | 44.42 | 1.98** | 19 | 7.72 | 2.46** | 33 | 17.46 | 1.89** | 36 | 19.24 | 1.87** |
| KIDNEY AND URETER | 19 | 6.23 | 3.05** | 8 | 1.10 | 7.25** | 5 | 2.52 | 1.99 | 6 | 2.61 | 2.30 |

Table 100. Subsequent primary sites with deficiencies

FIRST PRIMARY SITE - BLADDER

| SUBSEQUENT PRIMARY SITES | TOTAL<br>NUMBER OF PERSONS= 5996<br>PERSON-YRS OF OBSERVATION= 25775.7 | | | YEARS < 1<br>NUMBER OF PERSONS= 5996<br>PERSON-YRS OF OBSERVATION= 4823.7 | | | YEARS 1-5<br>NUMBER OF PERSONS= 4017<br>PERSON-YRS OF OBSERVATION= 10737.2 | | | YEARS > 5<br>NUMBER OF PERSONS= 1861<br>PERSON-YRS OF OBSERVATION= 10214.8 | | |
|---|---|---|---|---|---|---|---|---|---|---|---|---|
| | OBS | EXP | OBS/EXP | OBS | EXP | OBS/EXP | OBS | EXP | OBS/EXP | OBS | EXP | OBS/EXP |
| BLADDER | 1 | 19.62 | 0.05** | 0 | 3.49 | 0.0 | 0 | 7.83 | 0.0 | 1 | 8.30 | 0.12** |

Table 101. Histologic confirmation of multiple primary malignancies

FIRST PRIMARY SITE - BLADDER

| Subsequent primary site | Both tumors microscopically confirmed | | Only 1st tumor microscopically confirmed | | Only 2nd tumor microscopically confirmed | | Neither tumor microscopically confirmed | |
|---|---|---|---|---|---|---|---|---|
| | No. | % | No. | % | No. | % | No. | % |
| TONGUE | 8 | 88.9 | 1 | 11.1 | 0 | 0.0 | 0 | 0.0 |
| LUNG AND BRONCHUS | 34 | 77.3 | 9 | 20.5 | 1 | 2.3 | 0 | 0.0 |
| CORPUS UTERI | 4 | 100.0 | 0 | 0.0 | 0 | 0.0 | 0 | 0.0 |
| PROSTATE | 65 | 73.9 | 15 | 17.0 | 6 | 6.8 | 2 | 2.3 |
| KIDNEY AND URETER | 17 | 89.5 | 1 | 5.3 | 1 | 5.3 | 0 | 0.0 |

Table 102. Summary of site-group pairs with an excess of observed-over-expected subsequent primary malignancies: index tumors of the urinary system

I. Possibly artifact

Kidney/ureter ———————→ Soft tissue
Bladder ———————→ Corpus uteri

II. Possibly real

A. In organs within the same system

1. Same or paired organs

Kidney/ureter ←———————→ Kidney/ureter

2. Other

Kidney/ureter ←———————→ Bladder

B. In organs related structurally or functionally

Kidney/ureter ———————→ Prostate
Kidney/ureter ———————→ Testis
Bladder ———————→ Prostate

C. In organs apparently unrelated structurally or functionally

Bladder ———————→ Tongue
Bladder ———————→ Lung/bronchus

Table 103. Common metastatic sites for primary malignant tumors of the urinary system (HOLLAND and FREI, 1973; WILLIS, 1973; RUBIN, 1974)

| Anatomic location of the primary malignant tumor | Common metastatic sites |
|---|---|
| Kidney/ureter | Liver; lungs; regional lymph nodes; bone; thyroid; brain and spinal cord |
| Bladder | Regional lymph nodes; lung; liver; bone |

# Chapter 11

# Index Tumors of Lymphatic and Hematopoietic Tissues

Population Studied. 4,234 males and 3,289 females with malignant neoplasms of the lymphatic and hematopoietic tissues were followed for the subsequent development of independent primary malignant neoplasms; 161 such subsequent neoplasms were diagnosed. The cohort of individuals with a malignancy of the lymphatic and hematopoietic tissues contributed 17,240 person-years of observation.

Results. Detailed tabulations by site are presented in Tables 104-109. The reader is referred to Chapter 5 for a general explanation of the items in these tables.

Summary of Findings. Site-group pairs with a statistically significant excess of observed-over-expected subsequent primary cancers are categorized in Table 110 on the basis of possible relationships between the anatomic sites containing these cancers. In addition, possible artifactual relationships, based on a small number of cases and with no confirmation from other published reports, are emphasized.

Discussion. Table 111 presents the common metastatic sites for cancers arising within the lymphatic and hematopoietic tissues. These data, used in conjunction with the site-specific tabulations of the percentage of multiple primary malignancies with histologic confirmation, are useful in distinguishing real from artifactual associations.

The majority of site-group pairs noted in Table 110 are classified in category I as likely being spurious associations. Although patients with such multiple primary cancers have been previously reported (MOERTEL, 1966; BERG, 1967; NEWELL et al., 1974a), there is no confirmation from other studies that these particular combinations occur more frequently than expected on the basis of chance. In most instances, the number of observed cases illustrating these various associations are relatively few. Furthermore, the liver and pancreas are common sites for leukemic infiltration; since 100% microscopic confirmation was lacking in patients with both leukemia and a malignancy of either the liver/gall bladder or pancreas, the relationship suggested may be spurious. One study reported an increased risk of lung cancer in black males with leukemia (NEWELL et al., 1974a). This might add support to the association between leukemia and cancer of other/unspecified respiratory organs seen in the Connecticut tabulations. This relationship is based on only one observed case, however.

An analysis of the Memorial Hospital experience revealed that patients with lymphoma, myeloma, or leukemia have an increased risk of prostatic cancer (BERG, 1967). As in the present series, however, the excess of prostatic cancer would result if 1) patients dying with lymphoma, myeloma, or leukemia came to autopsy more frequently than individuals dying with other diseases, and 2) clinically silent prostatic cancer was discovered at the time of the autopsy examination.

The association between leukemia and prostatic cancer is intriguing in that it is bidirectional. Despite this, the relationship may have no biologic basis. Not all patients with this combination of malignancies had histologic confirmation of both lesions, and it is possible that leukemic infiltration of the prostate may be mistaken for prostatic cancer. The excess risk of kidney/ureteral cancer in leukemia patients may likewise be spurious as it is based on only five observed cases. Although unconfirmed by other studies, the combination of leukemia and cancer of several sites within the male genito-urinary system appears a number of times in the Connecticut material.

The reader may have preferred a finer definition of tumor types within the lymphatic and hematopoietic tissues (e.g., chronic lymphatic leukemia, chronic myeloid leukemia, etc.). More detailed analyses such as these were carried out, but they provided no new insights into the associations reported nor did they reveal new relationships. In the interest of brevity, these tabulations were not included in the monograph.

Investigations of subsequent cancers occurring among patients with malignancies of the lymphatic and hematopoietic tissues have revealed an increased risk of skin cancer (BERG, 1967; NEWELL et al., 1974a). Skin cancers (with the exception of malignant melanoma) were not included in the analysis of the Connecticut data. Such lesions may be treated on an outpatient basis, and not be reported to the Connecticut Tumor Registry.

As shown in Chapter 4, several studies have suggested that chemotherapy, radiation therapy or immune defects in patients with lymphoma, myeloma, or leukemia may play a role in the later development of other cancers (ROSNER, 1976; HODGIN and WEBSTER, 1976). The Connecticut data, on which the present study is based, do not provide enough detail concerning treatment to allow one to test these hypotheses relating to chemotherapy.

Table 104. Subsequent multiple primary malignancies in patients with an index malignant lymphoma or myeloma

FIRST PRIMARY SITE - LYMPHOMAS AND MYELOMA

| SUBSEQUENT PRIMARY SITES | TOTAL NUMBER OF PERSONS= 4223 PERSON-YRS OF OBSERVATION = 11539.0 | | | MALES NUMBER OF PERSONS= 2323 PERSON-YRS OF OBSERVATION = 6216.4 | | | FEMALES NUMBER OF PERSONS= 1900 PERSON-YRS OF OBSERVATION = 5322.6 | | |
|---|---|---|---|---|---|---|---|---|---|
| | OBS | EXP | OBS/EXP | OBS | EXP | OBS/EXP | OBS | EXP | OBS/EXP |
| LIP | 2 | 0.62 | 3.20 | 2 | 0.59 | 3.38 | 0 | 0.03 | 0.0 |
| TONGUE | 1 | 0.58 | 1.73 | 1 | 0.50 | 1.99 | 0 | 0.07 | 0.0 |
| SALIVARY GLAND | 0 | 0.20 | 0.0 | 0 | 0.12 | 0.0 | 0 | 0.08 | 0.0 |
| MOUTH | 1 | 0.73 | 1.38 | 1 | 0.61 | 1.64 | 0 | 0.12 | 0.0 |
| PHARYNX | 4 | 0.78 | 5.16* | 2 | 0.67 | 3.01 | 2 | 0.11 | 18.20* |
| ESOPHAGUS | 0 | 1.23 | 0.0 | 0 | 1.09 | 0.0 | 0 | 0.14 | 0.0 |
| STOMACH | 3 | 5.02 | 0.60 | 2 | 3.47 | 0.58 | 1 | 1.55 | 0.65 |
| SMALL INTESTINE | 0 | 0.22 | 0.0 | 0 | 0.13 | 0.0 | 0 | 0.10 | 0.0 |
| COLON | 7 | 7.85 | 0.89 | 3 | 4.16 | 0.72 | 4 | 3.69 | 1.08 |
| RECTUM | 3 | 4.39 | 0.68 | 1 | 2.77 | 0.36 | 2 | 1.61 | 1.24 |
| LIVER & BILIARY PASS | 1 | 1.49 | 0.67 | 0 | 0.76 | 0.0 | 1 | 0.73 | 1.36 |
| PANCREAS | 4 | 2.18 | 1.84 | 2 | 1.40 | 1.43 | 2 | 0.78 | 2.55 |
| NOSE AND SINUSES | 0 | 0.14 | 0.0 | 0 | 0.09 | 0.0 | 0 | 0.05 | 0.0 |
| LARYNX | 0 | 1.00 | 0.0 | 0 | 0.93 | 0.0 | 0 | 0.06 | 0.0 |
| LUNG AND BRONCHUS | 8 | 6.10 | 1.31 | 8 | 5.39 | 1.49 | 0 | 0.71 | 0.0 |
| OTHER RESP | 0 | 0.11 | 0.0 | 0 | 0.09 | 0.0 | 0 | 0.02 | 0.0 |
| BREAST | 7 | 7.00 | 1.00 | 0 | 0.10 | 0.0 | 7 | 6.91 | 1.01 |
| CERVIX UTERI | 5 | 2.24 | 2.23 | 0 | 0.0 | 0.0 | 5 | 2.24 | 2.23 |
| CORPUS UTERI | 0 | 1.52 | 0.0 | 0 | 0.0 | 0.0 | 0 | 1.52 | 0.0 |
| UTERUS,UNSPEC | 2 | 0.73 | 2.72 | 0 | 0.0 | 0.0 | 2 | 0.73 | 2.72 |
| OVARY | 0 | 1.43 | 0.0 | 0 | 0.0 | 0.0 | 0 | 1.43 | 0.0 |
| OTHER FEMALE GENITAL | 0 | 0.27 | 0.0 | 0 | 0.0 | 0.0 | 0 | 0.27 | 0.0 |
| PROSTATE | 9 | 5.84 | 1.54 | 9 | 5.84 | 1.54 | 0 | 0.0 | 0.0 |
| TESTIS | 2 | 0.18 | 11.22* | 2 | 0.18 | 11.22* | 0 | 0.0 | 0.0 |
| OTHER MALE GENITAL | 0 | 0.14 | 0.0 | 0 | 0.14 | 0.0 | 0 | 0.0 | 0.0 |
| KIDNEY AND URETER | 4 | 1.30 | 3.07 | 3 | 0.90 | 3.33 | 1 | 0.40 | 2.48 |
| BLADDER | 3 | 3.40 | 0.88 | 3 | 2.68 | 1.12 | 0 | 0.72 | 0.0 |
| MELANOMA OF SKIN | 1 | 0.55 | 1.81 | 1 | 0.28 | 3.52 | 0 | 0.27 | 0.0 |
| EYE | 0 | 0.13 | 0.0 | 0 | 0.07 | 0.0 | 0 | 0.05 | 0.0 |
| NERVOUS SYSTEM | 0 | 0.81 | 0.0 | 0 | 0.48 | 0.0 | 0 | 0.33 | 0.0 |
| THYROID | 1 | 0.37 | 2.67 | 0 | 0.12 | 0.0 | 1 | 0.25 | 4.00 |
| BONE | 0 | 0.19 | 0.0 | 0 | 0.11 | 0.0 | 0 | 0.08 | 0.0 |
| SOFT TISSUE | 2 | 0.48 | 4.20 | 1 | 0.28 | 3.62 | 1 | 0.20 | 5.01 |
| LYMPHOMAS & MYELOMA | 1 | 2.02 | 0.50 | 0 | 1.21 | 0.0 | 1 | 0.81 | 1.24 |
| LEUKEMIAS | 0 | 1.83 | 0.0 | 0 | 1.18 | 0.0 | 0 | 0.65 | 0.0 |
| OTHER SITES | 5 | 3.52 | 1.42 | 3 | 2.03 | 1.48 | 2 | 1.49 | 1.35 |
| TOTAL | 76 | 66.58 | 1.14 | 44 | 38.36 | 1.15 | 32 | 28.22 | 1.13 |

Table 105. Subsequent primary sites with excesses

FIRST PRIMARY SITE - LYMPHOMAS AND MYELOMA

| SUBSEQUENT PRIMARY SITES | TOTAL | | | YEARS < 1 | | | YEARS 1-5 | | | YEARS > 5 | | |
|---|---|---|---|---|---|---|---|---|---|---|---|---|
| | NUMBER OF PERSONS= 4223 PERSON-YRS OF OBSERVATION= 11539.0 | | | NUMBER OF PERSONS= 4223 PERSON-YRS OF OBSERVATION= 2975.1 | | | NUMBER OF PERSONS= 2261 PERSON-YRS OF OBSERVATION= 5115.4 | | | NUMBER OF PERSONS= 704 PERSON-YRS OF OBSERVATION= 3448.5 | | |
| | OBS | EXP | OBS/EXP | OBS | EXP | OBS/EXP | OBS | EXP | OBS/EXP | OBS | EXP | OBS/EXP |
| PHARYNX | 4 | 0.78 | 5.16* | 1 | 0.21 | 4.72 | 3 | 0.33 | 9.11** | 0 | 0.23 | 0.0 |
| PROSTATE | 9 | 5.84 | 1.54 | 6 | 1.57 | 3.81* | 2 | 2.35 | 0.85 | 1 | 1.91 | 0.52 |
| TESTIS | 2 | 0.18 | 11.22* | 1 | 0.04 | 22.76 | 1 | 0.08 | 12.40 | 0 | 0.05 | 0.0 |

Table 106. Histologic confirmation of multiple primary malignancies

FIRST PRIMARY SITE - LYMPHOMAS AND MYELOMA

| Subsequent primary site | Both tumors microscopically confirmed | | Only 1st tumor microscopically confirmed | | Only 2nd tumor microscopically confirmed | | Neither tumor microscopically confirmed | |
|---|---|---|---|---|---|---|---|---|
| | No. | % | No. | % | No. | % | No. | % |
| PHARYNX | 4 | 100.0 | 0 | 0.0 | 0 | 0.0 | 0 | 0.0 |
| PROSTATE | 9 | 100.0 | 0 | 0.0 | 0 | 0.0 | 0 | 0.0 |
| TESTIS | 2 | 100.0 | 0 | 0.0 | 0 | 0.0 | 0 | 0.0 |

Table 107. Subsequent multiple primary malignancies in patients with an index leukemia

FIRST PRIMARY SITE - LEUKEMIAS

| SUBSEQUENT PRIMARY SITES | TOTAL | | | MALES | | | FEMALES | | |
|---|---|---|---|---|---|---|---|---|---|
| | NUMBER OF PERSONS= 3300 PERSON-YRS OF OBSERVATION = 5701.3 | | | NUMBER OF PERSONS= 1911 PERSON-YRS OF OBSERVATION = 3340.2 | | | NUMBER OF PERSONS= 1389 PERSON-YRS OF OBSERVATION = 2361.2 | | |
| | OBS | EXP | OBS/EXP | OBS | EXP | OBS/EXP | OBS | EXP | OBS/EXP |
| LIP | 1 | 0.55 | 1.81 | 1 | 0.53 | 1.89 | 0 | 0.02 | 0.0 |
| TONGUE | 2 | 0.51 | 3.96 | 2 | 0.46 | 4.39 | 0 | 0.05 | 0.0 |
| SALIVARY GLAND | 0 | 0.16 | 0.0 | 0 | 0.10 | 0.0 | 0 | 0.05 | 0.0 |
| MOUTH | 1 | 0.64 | 1.56 | 0 | 0.55 | 0.0 | 1 | 0.09 | 11.60 |
| PHARYNX | 0 | 0.63 | 0.0 | 0 | 0.57 | 0.0 | 0 | 0.07 | 0.0 |
| ESOPHAGUS | 1 | 1.12 | 0.89 | 1 | 1.01 | 0.99 | 0 | 0.11 | 0.0 |
| STOMACH | 3 | 4.59 | 0.65 | 2 | 3.31 | 0.60 | 1 | 1.28 | 0.78 |
| SMALL INTESTINE | 0 | 0.19 | 0.0 | 0 | 0.12 | 0.0 | 0 | 0.07 | 0.0 |
| COLON | 10 | 6.88 | 1.45 | 6 | 4.05 | 1.48 | 4 | 2.82 | 1.42 |
| RECTUM | 3 | 3.78 | 0.79 | 2 | 2.59 | 0.77 | 1 | 1.19 | 0.84 |
| LIVER & BILIARY PASS | 4 | 1.32 | 3.02 | 2 | 0.73 | 2.74 | 2 | 0.59 | 3.37 |
| PANCREAS | 7 | 1.95 | 3.59** | 2 | 1.34 | 1.50 | 5 | 0.61 | 8.16** |
| NOSE AND SINUSES | 0 | 0.11 | 0.0 | 0 | 0.08 | 0.0 | 0 | 0.03 | 0.0 |
| LARYNX | 2 | 0.87 | 2.29 | 2 | 0.84 | 2.39 | 0 | 0.04 | 0.0 |
| LUNG AND BRONCHUS | 8 | 5.33 | 1.50 | 7 | 4.84 | 1.45 | 1 | 0.49 | 2.03 |
| OTHER RESP | 1 | 0.09 | 11.49 | 1 | 0.07 | 13.79 | 0 | 0.01 | 0.0 |
| BREAST | 3 | 4.38 | 0.69 | 0 | 0.09 | 0.0 | 3 | 4.29 | 0.70 |
| CERVIX UTERI | 2 | 0.97 | 2.06 | 0 | 0.0 | 0.0 | 2 | 0.97 | 2.06 |
| CORPUS UTERI | 0 | 0.93 | 0.0 | 0 | 0.0 | 0.0 | 0 | 0.93 | 0.0 |
| UTERUS,UNSPEC | 0 | 0.50 | 0.0 | 0 | 0.0 | 0.0 | 0 | 0.50 | 0.0 |
| OVARY | 1 | 0.85 | 1.18 | 0 | 0.0 | 0.0 | 1 | 0.85 | 1.18 |
| OTHER FEMALE GENITAL | 1 | 0.20 | 4.89 | 0 | 0.0 | 0.0 | 1 | 0.20 | 4.89 |
| PROSTATE | 18 | 6.19 | 2.91** | 18 | 6.19 | 2.91** | 0 | 0.0 | 0.0 |
| TESTIS | 1 | 0.08 | 12.97 | 1 | 0.08 | 12.97 | 0 | 0.0 | 0.0 |
| OTHER MALE GENITAL | 0 | 0.12 | 0.0 | 0 | 0.12 | 0.0 | 0 | 0.0 | 0.0 |
| KIDNEY AND URETER | 5 | 1.09 | 4.59* | 5 | 0.80 | 6.24** | 0 | 0.29 | 0.0 |
| BLADDER | 3 | 3.13 | 0.96 | 3 | 2.57 | 1.17 | 0 | 0.56 | 0.0 |
| MELANOMA OF SKIN | 1 | 0.34 | 2.93 | 1 | 0.20 | 5.05 | 0 | 0.14 | 0.0 |
| EYE | 0 | 0.10 | 0.0 | 0 | 0.06 | 0.0 | 0 | 0.04 | 0.0 |
| NERVOUS SYSTEM | 0 | 0.47 | 0.0 | 0 | 0.30 | 0.0 | 0 | 0.17 | 0.0 |
| THYROID | 0 | 0.24 | 0.0 | 0 | 0.10 | 0.0 | 0 | 0.14 | 0.0 |
| BONE | 0 | 0.14 | 0.0 | 0 | 0.09 | 0.0 | 0 | 0.06 | 0.0 |
| SOFT TISSUE | 2 | 0.36 | 5.63 | 2 | 0.24 | 8.45* | 0 | 0.12 | 0.0 |
| LYMPHOMAS & MYELOMA | 1 | 1.46 | 0.69 | 1 | 0.96 | 1.05 | 0 | 0.50 | 0.0 |
| LEUKEMIAS | 1 | 1.56 | 0.64 | 1 | 1.09 | 0.92 | 0 | 0.48 | 0.0 |
| OTHER SITES | 3 | 3.05 | 0.98 | 1 | 1.92 | 0.52 | 2 | 1.12 | 1.78 |
| TOTAL | 85 | 54.89 | 1.55** | 61 | 36.00 | 1.69** | 24 | 18.89 | 1.27 |

Table 108. Subsequent primary sites with excesses

FIRST PRIMARY SITE - LEUKEMIAS

| SUBSEQUENT PRIMARY SITES | TOTAL<br>NUMBER OF PERSONS= 3300<br>PERSON-YRS OF OBSERVATION= 5701.3 | | | YEARS < 1<br>NUMBER OF PERSONS= 3300<br>PERSON-YRS OF OBSERVATION= 1996.1 | | | YEARS 1-5<br>NUMBER OF PERSONS= 1396<br>PERSON-YRS OF OBSERVATION= 2726.2 | | | YEARS > 5<br>NUMBER OF PERSONS= 306<br>PERSON-YRS OF OBSERVATION= 979.1 | | |
|---|---|---|---|---|---|---|---|---|---|---|---|---|
| | OBS | EXP | OBS/EXP | OBS | EXP | OBS/EXP | OBS | EXP | OBS/EXP | OBS | EXP | OBS/EXP |
| LIVER & BILIARY PASS | 4 | 1.32 | 3.02 | 3 | 0.40 | 7.55* | 1 | 0.64 | 1.55 | 0 | 0.28 | 0.0 |
| PANCREAS | 7 | 1.95 | 3.59** | 3 | 0.58 | 5.20* | 2 | 0.94 | 2.12 | 2 | 0.43 | 4.63 |
| OTHER RESP | 1 | 0.09 | 11.49 | 0 | 0.03 | 0.0 | 0 | 0.04 | 0.0 | 1 | 0.02 | 53.99* |
| PROSTATE | 13 | 6.19 | 2.91** | 8 | 1.85 | 4.31** | 10 | 2.97 | 3.37** | 0 | 1.37 | 0.0 |
| KIDNEY AND URETER | 5 | 1.09 | 4.59* | 2 | 0.33 | 6.15 | 2 | 0.53 | 3.80 | 1 | 0.24 | 4.20 |
| SOFT TISSUE | 2 | 0.36 | 5.63 | 1 | 0.11 | 9.47 | 0 | 0.17 | 0.0 | 1 | 0.08 | 12.87 |

Table 109. Histologic confirmation of multiple primary malignancies

FIRST PRIMARY SITE - LEUKEMIAS

| Subsequent primary site | Both tumors microscopically confirmed | | Only 1st tumor microscopically confirmed | | Only 2nd tumor microscopically confirmed | | Neither tumor microscopically confirmed | |
|---|---|---|---|---|---|---|---|---|
| | No. | % | No. | % | No. | % | No. | % |
| LIVER & BILIARY PASS | 2 | 50.0 | 0 | 0.0 | 2 | 50.0 | 0 | 0.0 |
| PANCREAS | 3 | 42.9 | 4 | 57.1 | 0 | 0.0 | 0 | 0.0 |
| OTHER RESP | 1 | 100.0 | 0 | 0.0 | 0 | 0.0 | 0 | 0.0 |
| PROSTATE | 14 | 77.8 | 2 | 11.1 | 2 | 11.1 | 0 | 0.0 |
| KIDNEY AND URETER | 4 | 80.0 | 0 | 0.0 | 1 | 20.0 | 0 | 0.0 |
| SOFT TISSUE | 2 | 100.0 | 0 | 0.0 | 0 | 0.0 | 0 | 0.0 |

Table 110. Summary of site-group pairs with an excess of observed-over-expected subsequent primary malignancies: index malignancies of the lymphatic and hematopoietic tissues

I. Possibly artifact

- Lymphoma/myeloma ——→ Pharynx
- Lymphoma/myeloma ——→ Prostate
- Lymphoma/myeloma ——→ Testis
- Leukemia ——→ Liver/biliary passages
- Leukemia ——→ Pancreas
- Leukemia ——→ Other/unspecified respiratory
- Leukemia ——→ Soft tissue

II. Possibly real

A. In organs within the same system

None

B. In organs related structurally or functionally

None

C. In organs apparently unrelated structurally or functionally

- Leukemia ←——→ Prostate
- Leukemia ——→ Kidney/ureter

Table 111. Common metastatic sites for primary malignant tumors of lymphatic and hematopoietic tissues (HOLLAND and FREI, 1973; WILLIS, 1973; RUBIN, 1974)

| Anatomic location of the primary malignant tumor | Common metastatic sites |
|---|---|
| Lymphomas | Bone marrow; spleen; bone; liver; spinal cord |
| Leukemias | Lymph nodes; bone marrow; central nervous system (brain, pituitary, spinal cord, meninges); spleen; liver; pancreas; thyroid; salivary glands; gingiva; lung; skin; gastro-intestinal tract (anywhere from mouth to rectum); orbit |

# Chapter 12

# Index Tumors of Remaining and Ill-Defined Sites

Population Studied. 5,379 males and 5,419 females with cancer of the remaining and ill-defined sites were followed for the subsequent development of independent primary malignant neoplasms; 247 such subsequent neoplasms were discovered. The cohort of patients with cancer of the remaining and ill-defined sites contributed 28,391 person-years of observation.

Results. Detailed tabulations by site are presented in Tables 112-132. The reader is referred to Chapter 5 for a general explanation of the items in these tables.

Summary of Findings. Site-specific pairs with a statistically significant excess of observed-over-expected subsequent primary cancers are categorized in Table 133 on the basis of possible relationships between the anatomic sites containing these cancers. In addition, possible artifactual relationships, based on a small number of cases and with no confirmation from other published reports, are emphasized.

Discussion. Table 134 presents the common metastatic sites for cancers arising within the remaining sites. These data, used in conjunction with the site-specific tabulations of the percentage of multiple primary malignancies with histologic confirmation, are useful in distinguishing real from artifactual associations.

The large number of site-group pairs outlined in category I of Table 133 are thought to represent spurious associations. They are based on a relatively small number of observed cases, and are not confirmed by other investigations. Although the list appears to be quite long, the reader should bear in mind that a large number of sites comprise the group labeled "remaining and ill-defined sites." Tumors in these locations are relatively rare, and the observed number of cases is therefore quite small. Perhaps this also accounts for the lack of confirmation from other studies. One must accumulate a substantial population under observation to obtain sufficiently large numbers for statistical significance. Perhaps as this type of investigation is replicated with other data resources, evidence will emerge supporting a biologic mechanism for site-group pairs currently classified as artifactual. However, with a large number of sites in this last group, over 1,000 comparisons were made, and one might expect over 50 associations to be statistically significant by chance.

For relationships classified under category IIA, excess risks could be explained on the basis of the same or similar tissue being exposed to a common oncogenic agent(s). In patients with multiple malignant melanomas of the skin, it is obviously difficult to distinguish metastatic disease from a new primary malignancy. The presence of bilateral retinoblastoma of the eye is a well-documented phenomenon (KITCHIN and ELLSWORTH, 1974).

The excess risk of a bone malignancy in patients with a malignant neoplasm of the eye, although based on one observed case, has been reported. Retinoblastoma patients treated with radiation are at increased risk for the subsequent development of osteosarcoma in areas both within and far removed from the field of radiation (JENSEN and MILLER, 1971; KITCHIN and ELLSWORTH, 1974).

The association between brain and breast is based on five cases, and includes only neoplasms of the brain specified as malignant. Since both benign and malignant central nervous system neoplasms are reportable to the Connecticut Tumor Registry, a special study was carried out concerning the relationship between central nervous system neoplasms (both benign and malignant) and primary malignancies of other sites. A bidirectional association was discovered between meningioma and breast cancer in women (SCHOENBERG et al., 1975). This result has not yet been confirmed by other studies, but raises several possible etiologic clues when considered with other epidemiologic features of meningiomas. First, meningioma is the only common intracranial neoplasm with a higher incidence in females (SCHOENBERG et al., 1976); second, the abrupt onset of clinical symptoms or enlargement of meningioma during pregnancy has been reported (MICHELSEN and NEW, 1969).

The excess risk of leukemia in patients with thyroid cancer probably represents the leukemogenic effects of radiation used to treat carcinoma of the thyroid. This relationship is well-established in the literature (MOERTEL, 1966; JABLON, 1975). Note that the excess risk is concentrated in the period 1-5 years after diagnosis of the thyroid cancer. This is consistent with the reported 3-1/2-year average interval between initiation of therapy for thyroid cancer and the diagnosis of leukemia (MOERTEL, 1966).

The link between soft-tissue malignancies and colon cancer may represent a variant of Gardner's syndrome in which familial polyposis of the colon is associated with osteomas, fibromas, lipomas, and epidermal cysts (GARDNER and RICHARDS, 1953).

The excess risk of breast cancer in patients with malignant melanoma of the skin is based on 9 individuals. In each patient, both malignant neoplasms were verified microscopically; furthermore, malignant melanoma only rarely metastasizes to the breast (JOCHIMSEN and BROWN, 1976). VAISMAN et al. (1976) also reported this same association between breast cancer and malignant melanoma, although their analysis was based on the experience of patients seen at a particular clinic. The relationship has additional support from the findings of social data collected as part of the United States Third National Cancer Survey. Unexpectedly both breast cancer and malignant melanoma were positively correlated with alcohol consumption (WILLIAMS, 1976). The author of that report hypothetically linked these cancers to the secretion of prolactin and melanocyte-stimulating hormone, thought to be the result of alcohol-induced stimulation of the pituitary gland.

Table 112. Subsequent multiple primary malignancies in patients with an index malignant melanoma of the skin

FIRST PRIMARY SITE - MALIGNANT MELANOMA OF SKIN

| SUBSEQUENT PRIMARY SITES | TOTAL NUMBER OF PERSONS= 1347 PERSON-YRS OF OBSERVATION = 5344.8 | | | MALES NUMBER OF PERSONS= 636 PERSON-YRS OF OBSERVATION = 2158.6 | | | FEMALES NUMBER OF PERSONS= 711 PERSON-YRS OF OBSERVATION = 3186.2 | | |
|---|---|---|---|---|---|---|---|---|---|
| | OBS | EXP | OBS/EXP | OBS | EXP | OBS/EXP | OBS | EXP | OBS/EXP |
| LIP | 1 | 0.26 | 3.85 | 1 | 0.23 | 4.26 | 0 | 0.03 | 0.0 |
| TONGUE | 0 | 0.24 | 0.0 | 0 | 0.19 | 0.0 | 0 | 0.05 | 0.0 |
| SALIVARY GLAND | 1 | 0.10 | 9.52 | 1 | 0.05 | 20.99 | 0 | 0.06 | 0.0 |
| MOUTH | 1 | 0.32 | 3.12 | 0 | 0.23 | 0.0 | 1 | 0.09 | 11.30 |
| PHARYNX | 0 | 0.32 | 0.0 | 0 | 0.24 | 0.0 | 0 | 0.08 | 0.0 |
| ESOPHAGUS | 2 | 0.50 | 3.99 | 1 | 0.39 | 2.57 | 1 | 0.11 | 8.96 |
| STOMACH | 1 | 2.56 | 0.39 | 1 | 1.33 | 0.75 | 0 | 1.23 | 0.0 |
| SMALL INTESTINE | 0 | 0.12 | 0.0 | 0 | 0.05 | 0.0 | 0 | 0.07 | 0.0 |
| COLON | 4 | 4.28 | 0.93 | 1 | 1.56 | 0.64 | 3 | 2.72 | 1.10 |
| RECTUM | 5 | 2.18 | 2.29 | 4 | 1.01 | 3.95* | 1 | 1.17 | 0.86 |
| LIVER & BILIARY PASS | 1 | 0.86 | 1.17 | 1 | 0.29 | 3.40 | 0 | 0.56 | 0.0 |
| PANCREAS | 2 | 1.10 | 1.81 | 1 | 0.52 | 1.92 | 1 | 0.58 | 1.72 |
| NOSE AND SINUSES | 0 | 0.07 | 0.0 | 0 | 0.03 | 0.0 | 0 | 0.03 | 0.0 |
| LARYNX | 0 | 0.39 | 0.0 | 0 | 0.34 | 0.0 | 0 | 0.04 | 0.0 |
| LUNG AND BRONCHUS | 3 | 2.38 | 1.26 | 3 | 1.87 | 1.61 | 0 | 0.51 | 0.0 |
| OTHER RESP | 0 | 0.05 | 0.0 | 0 | 0.03 | 0.0 | 0 | 0.02 | 0.0 |
| BREAST | 9 | 4.90 | 1.84 | 0 | 0.04 | 0.0 | 9 | 4.86 | 1.85 |
| CERVIX UTERI | 1 | 1.45 | 0.69 | 0 | 0.0 | 0.0 | 1 | 1.45 | 0.69 |
| CORPUS UTERI | 2 | 1.02 | 1.97 | 0 | 0.0 | 0.0 | 2 | 1.02 | 1.97 |
| UTERUS,UNSPEC | 2 | 0.53 | 3.78 | 0 | 0.0 | 0.0 | 2 | 0.53 | 3.78 |
| OVARY | 1 | 0.96 | 1.04 | 0 | 0.0 | 0.0 | 1 | 0.96 | 1.04 |
| OTHER FEMALE GENITAL | 1 | 0.20 | 4.99 | 0 | 0.0 | 0.0 | 1 | 0.20 | 4.99 |
| PROSTATE | 2 | 2.35 | 0.85 | 2 | 2.35 | 0.85 | 0 | 0.0 | 0.0 |
| TESTIS | 0 | 0.07 | 0.0 | 0 | 0.07 | 0.0 | 0 | 0.0 | 0.0 |
| OTHER MALE GENITAL | 0 | 0.06 | 0.0 | 0 | 0.06 | 0.0 | 0 | 0.0 | 0.0 |
| KIDNEY AND URETER | 2 | 0.60 | 3.31 | 2 | 0.32 | 6.28 | 0 | 0.29 | 0.0 |
| BLADDER | 1 | 1.54 | 0.65 | 1 | 0.99 | 1.01 | 0 | 0.54 | 0.0 |
| MELANOMA OF SKIN | 6 | 0.29 | 20.42** | 6 | 0.11 | 52.74** | 0 | 0.18 | 0.0 |
| EYE | 0 | 0.07 | 0.0 | 0 | 0.03 | 0.0 | 0 | 0.04 | 0.0 |
| NERVOUS SYSTEM | 1 | 0.38 | 2.67 | 1 | 0.16 | 6.10 | 0 | 0.21 | 0.0 |
| THYROID | 0 | 0.22 | 0.0 | 0 | 0.05 | 0.0 | 0 | 0.18 | 0.0 |
| BONE | 0 | 0.10 | 0.0 | 0 | 0.04 | 0.0 | 0 | 0.06 | 0.0 |
| SOFT TISSUE | 1 | 0.24 | 4.19 | 0 | 0.11 | 0.0 | 1 | 0.13 | 7.54 |
| LYMPHOMAS & MYELOMA | 2 | 0.96 | 2.08 | 0 | 0.43 | 0.0 | 2 | 0.54 | 3.73 |
| LEUKEMIAS | 0 | 0.88 | 0.0 | 0 | 0.42 | 0.0 | 0 | 0.46 | 0.0 |
| OTHER SITES | 6 | 1.85 | 3.24* | 3 | 0.76 | 3.93 | 3 | 1.09 | 2.75 |
| TOTAL | 58 | 34.39 | 1.69** | 29 | 14.32 | 2.03** | 29 | 20.07 | 1.45 |

Table 113. Subsequent primary sites with excesses

FIRST PRIMARY SITE - MALIGNANT MELANOMA OF SKIN

| | TOTAL | | | YEARS < 1 | | | YEARS 1-5 | | | YEARS > 5 | | |
|---|---|---|---|---|---|---|---|---|---|---|---|---|
| | NUMBER OF PERSONS= 1347 PERSON-YRS OF OBSERVATION= 5344.8 | | | NUMBER OF PERSONS= 1347 PERSON-YRS OF OBSERVATION= 1151.9 | | | NUMBER OF PERSONS= 989 PERSON-YRS OF OBSERVATION= 2385.8 | | | NUMBER OF PERSONS= 352 PERSON-YRS OF OBSERVATION= 1807.1 | | |
| SUBSEQUENT PRIMARY SITES | OBS | EXP | OBS/EXP | OBS | EXP | OBS/EXP | OBS | EXP | OBS/EXP | OBS | EXP | OBS/EXP |
| SALIVARY GLAND | 1 | 0.10 | 9.52 | 1 | 0.02 | 45.45* | 0 | 0.04 | 0.0 | 0 | 0.04 | 0.0 |
| ESOPHAGUS | 2 | 0.50 | 3.99 | 0 | 0.12 | 0.0 | 2 | 0.22 | 9.26* | 0 | 0.17 | 0.0 |
| RECTUM | 5 | 2.18 | 2.29 | 1 | 0.46 | 2.18 | 4 | 0.92 | 4.35* | 0 | 0.80 | 0.0 |
| BREAST | 9 | 4.90 | 1.84 | 0 | 0.86 | 0.0 | 3 | 2.06 | 1.46 | 6 | 1.97 | 3.05* |
| MELANOMA OF SKIN | 6 | 0.29 | 20.42** | 6 | 0.06 | 95.65** | 0 | 0.13 | 0.0 | 0 | 0.11 | 0.0 |
| OTHER SITES | 6 | 1.85 | 3.24* | 2 | 0.37 | 5.42 | 2 | 0.75 | 2.66 | 2 | 0.73 | 2.73 |

Table 114. Histologic confirmation of multiple primary malignancies

FIRST PRIMARY SITE - MALIGNANT MELANOMA OF SKIN

| Subsequent primary site | Both tumors microscopically confirmed | | Only 1st tumor microscopically confirmed | | Only 2nd tumor microscopically confirmed | | Neither tumor microscopically confirmed | |
|---|---|---|---|---|---|---|---|---|
| | No. | % | No. | % | No. | % | No. | % |
| SALIVARY GLAND | 1 | 100.0 | 0 | 0.0 | 0 | 0.0 | 0 | 0.0 |
| ESOPHAGUS | 2 | 100.0 | 0 | 0.0 | 0 | 0.0 | 0 | 0.0 |
| RECTUM | 4 | 80.0 | 1 | 20.0 | 0 | 0.0 | 0 | 0.0 |
| BREAST | 9 | 100.0 | 0 | 0.0 | 0 | 0.0 | 0 | 0.0 |
| MELANOMA OF SKIN | 6 | 100.0 | 0 | 0.0 | 0 | 0.0 | 0 | 0.0 |
| OTHER SITES | 4 | 66.7 | 2 | 33.3 | 0 | 0.0 | 0 | 0.0 |

Table 115. Subsequent multiple primary malignancies in patients with an index malignant tumor of the eye

FIRST PRIMARY SITE - EYE

| SUBSEQUENT PRIMARY SITES | TOTAL | | | MALES | | | FEMALES | | |
|---|---|---|---|---|---|---|---|---|---|
| | NUMBER OF PERSONS= 386 PERSON-YRS OF OBSERVATION = 2491.0 | | | NUMBER OF PERSONS= 200 PERSON-YRS OF OBSERVATION = 1188.8 | | | NUMBER OF PERSONS= 186 PERSON-YRS OF OBSERVATION = 1302.2 | | |
| | OBS | EXP | OBS/EXP | OBS | EXP | OBS/EXP | OBS | EXP | OBS/EXP |
| LIP | 0 | 0.17 | 0.0 | 0 | 0.16 | 0.0 | 0 | 0.01 | 0.0 |
| TONGUE | 0 | 0.15 | 0.0 | 0 | 0.13 | 0.0 | 0 | 0.02 | 0.0 |
| SALIVARY GLAND | 0 | 0.05 | 0.0 | 0 | 0.03 | 0.0 | 0 | 0.02 | 0.0 |
| MOUTH | 0 | 0.19 | 0.0 | 0 | 0.16 | 0.0 | 0 | 0.03 | 0.0 |
| PHARYNX | 0 | 0.19 | 0.0 | 0 | 0.16 | 0.0 | 0 | 0.03 | 0.0 |
| ESOPHAGUS | 0 | 0.33 | 0.0 | 0 | 0.29 | 0.0 | 0 | 0.04 | 0.0 |
| STOMACH | 1 | 1.49 | 0.67 | 1 | 1.00 | 1.00 | 0 | 0.49 | 0.0 |
| SMALL INTESTINE | 0 | 0.06 | 0.0 | 0 | 0.04 | 0.0 | 0 | 0.03 | 0.0 |
| COLON | 1 | 2.21 | 0.45 | 1 | 1.14 | 0.88 | 0 | 1.07 | 0.0 |
| RECTUM | 2 | 1.21 | 1.66 | 1 | 0.74 | 1.35 | 1 | 0.46 | 2.16 |
| LIVER & BILIARY PASS | 1 | 0.44 | 2.25 | 1 | 0.22 | 4.63 | 0 | 0.23 | 0.0 |
| PANCREAS | 1 | 0.60 | 1.67 | 0 | 0.37 | 0.0 | 1 | 0.23 | 4.41 |
| NOSE AND SINUSES | 0 | 0.03 | 0.0 | 0 | 0.02 | 0.0 | 0 | 0.01 | 0.0 |
| LARYNX | 0 | 0.24 | 0.0 | 0 | 0.23 | 0.0 | 0 | 0.01 | 0.0 |
| LUNG AND BRONCHUS | 3 | 1.46 | 2.06 | 3 | 1.27 | 2.37 | 0 | 0.19 | 0.0 |
| OTHER RESP | 0 | 0.03 | 0.0 | 0 | 0.02 | 0.0 | 0 | 0.01 | 0.0 |
| BREAST | 1 | 1.83 | 0.55 | 0 | 0.02 | 0.0 | 1 | 1.81 | 0.55 |
| CERVIX UTERI | 1 | 0.47 | 2.12 | 0 | 0.0 | 0.0 | 1 | 0.47 | 2.12 |
| CORPUS UTERI | 0 | 0.38 | 0.0 | 0 | 0.0 | 0.0 | 0 | 0.38 | 0.0 |
| UTERUS,UNSPEC | 1 | 0.21 | 4.66 | 0 | 0.0 | 0.0 | 1 | 0.21 | 4.66 |
| OVARY | 0 | 0.36 | 0.0 | 0 | 0.0 | 0.0 | 0 | 0.36 | 0.0 |
| OTHER FEMALE GENITAL | 0 | 0.08 | 0.0 | 0 | 0.0 | 0.0 | 0 | 0.08 | 0.0 |
| PROSTATE | 1 | 1.77 | 0.57 | 1 | 1.77 | 0.57 | 0 | 0.0 | 0.0 |
| TESTIS | 0 | 0.02 | 0.0 | 0 | 0.02 | 0.0 | 0 | 0.0 | 0.0 |
| OTHER MALE GENITAL | 0 | 0.04 | 0.0 | 0 | 0.04 | 0.0 | 0 | 0.0 | 0.0 |
| KIDNEY AND URETER | 0 | 0.33 | 0.0 | 0 | 0.22 | 0.0 | 0 | 0.11 | 0.0 |
| BLADDER | 0 | 0.92 | 0.0 | 0 | 0.71 | 0.0 | 0 | 0.22 | 0.0 |
| MELANOMA OF SKIN | 1 | 0.12 | 8.25 | 1 | 0.06 | 17.00 | 0 | 0.06 | 0.0 |
| EYE | 1 | 0.04 | 27.00 | 1 | 0.02 | 49.86* | 0 | 0.02 | 0.0 |
| NERVOUS SYSTEM | 0 | 0.17 | 0.0 | 0 | 0.09 | 0.0 | 0 | 0.08 | 0.0 |
| THYROID | 0 | 0.09 | 0.0 | 0 | 0.03 | 0.0 | 0 | 0.06 | 0.0 |
| BONE | 1 | 0.05 | 19.41 | 1 | 0.03 | 35.29 | 0 | 0.02 | 0.0 |
| SOFT TISSUE | 0 | 0.11 | 0.0 | 0 | 0.07 | 0.0 | 0 | 0.05 | 0.0 |
| LYMPHOMAS & MYELOMA | 2 | 0.47 | 4.30 | 2 | 0.26 | 7.56 | 0 | 0.20 | 0.0 |
| LEUKEMIAS | 2 | 0.49 | 4.12 | 1 | 0.30 | 3.32 | 1 | 0.18 | 5.45 |
| OTHER SITES | 2 | 0.98 | 2.05 | 1 | 0.54 | 1.84 | 1 | 0.43 | 2.30 |
| TOTAL | 22 | 17.78 | 1.24 | 15 | 10.14 | 1.48 | 7 | 7.64 | 0.92 |

Table 116. Subsequent primary sites with excesses

FIRST PRIMARY SITE - EYE

| SUBSEQUENT PRIMARY SITES | TOTAL<br>NUMBER OF PERSONS= 386<br>PERSON-YRS OF OBSERVATION= 2491.0 | | | YEARS < 1<br>NUMBER OF PERSONS= 386<br>PERSON-YRS OF OBSERVATION= 355.0 | | | YEARS 1-5<br>NUMBER OF PERSONS= 332<br>PERSON-YRS OF OBSERVATION= 952.7 | | | YEARS > 5<br>NUMBER OF PERSONS= 172<br>PERSON-YRS OF OBSERVATION= 1183.3 | | |
|---|---|---|---|---|---|---|---|---|---|---|---|---|
| | OBS | EXP | OBS/EXP | OBS | EXP | OBS/EXP | OBS | EXP | OBS/EXP | OBS | EXP | OBS/EXP |
| EYE | 1 | 0.04 | 27.00 | 0 | 0.01 | 0.0 | 1 | 0.01 | 72.69* | 0 | 0.02 | 0.0 |
| BONE | 1 | 0.05 | 19.41 | 0 | 0.01 | 0.0 | 0 | 0.02 | 0.0 | 1 | 0.03 | 39.53* |

Table 117. Histologic confirmation of multiple primary malignancies

FIRST PRIMARY SITE - EYE

| Subsequent primary site | Both tumors microscopically confirmed | | Only 1st tumor microscopically confirmed | | Only 2nd tumor microscopically confirmed | | Neither tumor microscopically confirmed | |
|---|---|---|---|---|---|---|---|---|
| | No. | % | No. | % | No. | % | No. | % |
| EYE | 1 | 100.0 | 0 | 0.0 | 0 | 0.0 | 0 | 0.0 |
| BONE | 1 | 100.0 | 0 | 0.0 | 0 | 0.0 | 0 | 0.0 |

Table 118. Subsequent multiple primary malignancies in patients with an index malignant tumor of the brain and nervous system

FIRST PRIMARY SITE - BRAIN AND NERVOUS SYSTEM

| SUBSEQUENT PRIMARY SITES | TOTAL NUMBER OF PERSONS= 1747 PERSON-YRS OF OBSERVATION = 3611.5 | | | MALES NUMBER OF PERSONS= 990 PERSON-YRS OF OBSERVATION = 1934.3 | | | FEMALES NUMBER OF PERSONS= 757 PERSON-YRS OF OBSERVATION = 1677.2 | | |
|---|---|---|---|---|---|---|---|---|---|
| | OBS | EXP | OBS/EXP | OBS | EXP | OBS/EXP | OBS | EXP | OBS/EXP |
| LIP | 0 | 0.10 | 0.0 | 0 | 0.09 | 0.0 | 0 | 0.00 | 0.0 |
| TONGUE | 0 | 0.10 | 0.0 | 0 | 0.08 | 0.0 | 0 | 0.01 | 0.0 |
| SALIVARY GLAND | 0 | 0.04 | 0.0 | 0 | 0.02 | 0.0 | 0 | 0.01 | 0.0 |
| MOUTH | 0 | 0.12 | 0.0 | 0 | 0.10 | 0.0 | 0 | 0.02 | 0.0 |
| PHARYNX | 0 | 0.13 | 0.0 | 0 | 0.11 | 0.0 | 0 | 0.02 | 0.0 |
| ESOPHAGUS | 0 | 0.19 | 0.0 | 0 | 0.17 | 0.0 | 0 | 0.02 | 0.0 |
| STOMACH | 2 | 0.71 | 2.80 | 1 | 0.50 | 1.99 | 1 | 0.21 | 4.73 |
| SMALL INTESTINE | 0 | 0.04 | 0.0 | 0 | 0.02 | 0.0 | 0 | 0.02 | 0.0 |
| COLON | 3 | 1.17 | 2.56 | 2 | 0.60 | 3.31 | 1 | 0.57 | 1.77 |
| RECTUM | 0 | 0.69 | 0.0 | 0 | 0.42 | 0.0 | 0 | 0.27 | 0.0 |
| LIVER & BILIARY PASS | 0 | 0.21 | 0.0 | 0 | 0.11 | 0.0 | 0 | 0.10 | 0.0 |
| PANCREAS | 0 | 0.32 | 0.0 | 0 | 0.21 | 0.0 | 0 | 0.11 | 0.0 |
| NOSE AND SINUSES | 0 | 0.02 | 0.0 | 0 | 0.01 | 0.0 | 0 | 0.01 | 0.0 |
| LARYNX | 0 | 0.18 | 0.0 | 0 | 0.17 | 0.0 | 0 | 0.01 | 0.0 |
| LUNG AND BRONCHUS | 1 | 1.09 | 0.92 | 1 | 0.97 | 1.03 | 0 | 0.12 | 0.0 |
| OTHER RESP | 0 | 0.02 | 0.0 | 0 | 0.02 | 0.0 | 0 | 0.01 | 0.0 |
| BREAST | 5 | 1.37 | 3.64* | 0 | 0.02 | 0.0 | 5 | 1.36 | 3.68* |
| CERVIX UTERI | 0 | 0.54 | 0.0 | 0 | 0.0 | 0.0 | 0 | 0.54 | 0.0 |
| CORPUS UTERI | 1 | 0.31 | 3.24 | 0 | 0.0 | 0.0 | 1 | 0.31 | 3.24 |
| UTERUS,UNSPEC | 0 | 0.14 | 0.0 | 0 | 0.0 | 0.0 | 0 | 0.14 | 0.0 |
| OVARY | 1 | 0.30 | 3.32 | 0 | 0.0 | 0.0 | 1 | 0.30 | 3.32 |
| OTHER FEMALE GENITAL | 0 | 0.04 | 0.0 | 0 | 0.0 | 0.0 | 0 | 0.04 | 0.0 |
| PROSTATE | 3 | 0.61 | 4.94* | 3 | 0.61 | 4.94* | 0 | 0.0 | 0.0 |
| TESTIS | 0 | 0.05 | 0.0 | 0 | 0.05 | 0.0 | 0 | 0.0 | 0.0 |
| OTHER MALE GENITAL | 0 | 0.02 | 0.0 | 0 | 0.02 | 0.0 | 0 | 0.0 | 0.0 |
| KIDNEY AND URETER | 2 | 0.23 | 8.73* | 2 | 0.16 | 12.67* | 0 | 0.07 | 0.0 |
| BLADDER | 0 | 0.50 | 0.0 | 0 | 0.40 | 0.0 | 0 | 0.10 | 0.0 |
| MELANOMA OF SKIN | 1 | 0.12 | 8.45 | 0 | 0.06 | 0.0 | 1 | 0.06 | 16.97 |
| EYE | 0 | 0.03 | 0.0 | 0 | 0.01 | 0.0 | 0 | 0.01 | 0.0 |
| NERVOUS SYSTEM | 0 | 0.20 | 0.0 | 0 | 0.12 | 0.0 | 0 | 0.08 | 0.0 |
| THYROID | 2 | 0.08 | 26.52** | 1 | 0.02 | 40.51* | 1 | 0.05 | 19.71 |
| BONE | 0 | 0.04 | 0.0 | 0 | 0.03 | 0.0 | 0 | 0.02 | 0.0 |
| SOFT TISSUE | 0 | 0.10 | 0.0 | 0 | 0.06 | 0.0 | 0 | 0.04 | 0.0 |
| LYMPHOMAS & MYELOMA | 2 | 0.39 | 5.11 | 0 | 0.23 | 0.0 | 2 | 0.16 | 12.73* |
| LEUKEMIAS | 1 | 0.33 | 3.03 | 1 | 0.21 | 4.81 | 0 | 0.12 | 0.0 |
| OTHER SITES | 2 | 0.56 | 3.60 | 2 | 0.33 | 6.10 | 0 | 0.23 | 0.0 |
| TOTAL | 26 | 11.09 | 2.34** | 13 | 5.94 | 2.19* | 13 | 5.15 | 2.52** |

Table 119. Subsequent primary sites with excesses

FIRST PRIMARY SITE - BRAIN AND NERVOUS SYSTEM

| SUBSEQUENT PRIMARY SITES | TOTAL | | | YEARS < 1 | | | YEARS 1-5 | | | YEARS > 5 | | |
|---|---|---|---|---|---|---|---|---|---|---|---|---|
| | NUMBER OF PERSONS= 1747 PERSON-YRS OF OBSERVATION= 3611.5 | | | NUMBER OF PERSONS= 1747 PERSON-YRS OF OBSERVATION= 1003.2 | | | NUMBER OF PERSONS= 618 PERSON-YRS OF OBSERVATION= 1418.8 | | | NUMBER OF PERSONS= 221 PERSON-YRS OF OBSERVATION= 1189.4 | | |
| | OBS | EXP | OBS/EXP | OBS | EXP | OBS/EXP | OBS | EXP | OBS/EXP | OBS | EXP | OBS/EXP |
| BREAST | 5 | 1.37 | 3.64* | 1 | 0.38 | 2.66 | 3 | 0.51 | 5.90* | 1 | 0.49 | 2.04 |
| PROSTATE | 3 | 0.61 | 4.94* | 2 | 0.18 | 11.33* | 0 | 0.16 | 0.0 | 1 | 0.27 | 3.72 |
| KIDNEY AND URETER | 2 | 0.23 | 8.73* | 2 | 0.07 | 28.20** | 0 | 0.08 | 0.0 | 0 | 0.08 | 0.0 |
| THYROID | 2 | 0.08 | 26.52** | 1 | 0.02 | 49.15* | 0 | 0.03 | 0.0 | 1 | 0.03 | 35.76 |
| LYMPHOMAS & MYELOMA | 2 | 0.39 | 5.11 | 1 | 0.11 | 8.85 | 1 | 0.13 | 7.50 | 0 | 0.15 | 0.0 |

Table 120. Histologic confirmation of multiple primary malignancies

FIRST PRIMARY SITE - BRAIN AND NERVOUS SYSTEM

| Subsequent primary site | Both tumors microscopically confirmed | | Only 1st tumor microscopically confirmed | | Only 2nd tumor microscopically confirmed | | Neither tumor microscopically confirmed | |
|---|---|---|---|---|---|---|---|---|
| | No. | % | No. | % | No. | % | No. | % |
| BREAST | 3 | 60.0 | 0 | 0.0 | 2 | 40.0 | 0 | 0.0 |
| PROSTATE | 1 | 33.3 | 0 | 0.0 | 1 | 33.3 | 1 | 33.3 |
| KIDNEY AND URETER | 1 | 50.0 | 1 | 50.0 | 0 | 0.0 | 0 | 0.0 |
| THYROID | 2 | 100.0 | 0 | 0.0 | 0 | 0.0 | 0 | 0.0 |
| LYMPHOMAS & MYELOMA | 0 | 0.0 | 0 | 0.0 | 2 | 100.0 | 0 | 0.0 |

Table 121. Subsequent multiple primary malignancies in patients with an index malignant tumor of the thyroid

FIRST PRIMARY SITE - THYROID

| SUBSEQUENT PRIMARY SITES | TOTAL | | | MALES | | | FEMALES | | |
|---|---|---|---|---|---|---|---|---|---|
| | NUMBER OF PERSONS= 863 | | | NUMBER OF PERSONS= 205 | | | NUMBER OF PERSONS= 658 | | |
| | PERSON-YRS OF OBSERVATION = 4428.2 | | | PERSON-YRS OF OBSERVATION = 899.0 | | | PERSON-YRS OF OBSERVATION = 3529.2 | | |
| | OBS | EXP | OBS/EXP | OBS | EXP | OBS/EXP | OBS | EXP | OBS/EXP |
| LIP | 1 | 0.11 | 9.21 | 0 | 0.09 | 0.0 | 1 | 0.02 | 55.17* |
| TONGUE | 0 | 0.12 | 0.0 | 0 | 0.08 | 0.0 | 0 | 0.05 | 0.0 |
| SALIVARY GLAND | 0 | 0.07 | 0.0 | 0 | 0.02 | 0.0 | 0 | 0.05 | 0.0 |
| MOUTH | 0 | 0.16 | 0.0 | 0 | 0.10 | 0.0 | 0 | 0.07 | 0.0 |
| PHARYNX | 0 | 0.17 | 0.0 | 0 | 0.11 | 0.0 | 0 | 0.07 | 0.0 |
| ESOPHAGUS | 0 | 0.25 | 0.0 | 0 | 0.17 | 0.0 | 0 | 0.08 | 0.0 |
| STOMACH | 0 | 1.34 | 0.0 | 0 | 0.51 | 0.0 | 0 | 0.83 | 0.0 |
| SMALL INTESTINE | 0 | 0.08 | 0.0 | 0 | 0.02 | 0.0 | 0 | 0.06 | 0.0 |
| COLON | 3 | 2.67 | 1.13 | 0 | 0.63 | 0.0 | 3 | 2.03 | 1.48 |
| RECTUM | 5 | 1.32 | 3.78* | 0 | 0.42 | 0.0 | 5 | 0.90 | 5.54** |
| LIVER & BILIARY PASS | 0 | 0.50 | 0.0 | 0 | 0.12 | 0.0 | 0 | 0.38 | 0.0 |
| PANCREAS | 1 | 0.63 | 1.58 | 0 | 0.22 | 0.0 | 1 | 0.42 | 2.39 |
| NOSE AND SINUSES | 0 | 0.04 | 0.0 | 0 | 0.01 | 0.0 | 0 | 0.03 | 0.0 |
| LARYNX | 2 | 0.20 | 10.14* | 0 | 0.15 | 0.0 | 2 | 0.04 | 45.04** |
| LUNG AND BRONCHUS | 1 | 1.33 | 0.75 | 0 | 0.91 | 0.0 | 1 | 0.42 | 2.36 |
| OTHER RESP | 0 | 0.03 | 0.0 | 0 | 0.01 | 0.0 | 0 | 0.02 | 0.0 |
| BREAST | 8 | 4.43 | 1.80 | 0 | 0.02 | 0.0 | 8 | 4.42 | 1.81 |
| CERVIX UTERI | 1 | 1.67 | 0.60 | 0 | 0.0 | 0.0 | 1 | 1.67 | 0.60 |
| CORPUS UTERI | 3 | 0.96 | 3.14 | 0 | 0.0 | 0.0 | 3 | 0.96 | 3.14 |
| UTERUS,UNSPEC | 0 | 0.43 | 0.0 | 0 | 0.0 | 0.0 | 0 | 0.43 | 0.0 |
| OVARY | 0 | 0.91 | 0.0 | 0 | 0.0 | 0.0 | 0 | 0.91 | 0.0 |
| OTHER FEMALE GENITAL | 0 | 0.15 | 0.0 | 0 | 0.0 | 0.0 | 0 | 0.15 | 0.0 |
| PROSTATE | 1 | 0.89 | 1.12 | 1 | 0.89 | 1.12 | 0 | 0.0 | 0.0 |
| TESTIS | 0 | 0.02 | 0.0 | 0 | 0.02 | 0.0 | 0 | 0.0 | 0.0 |
| OTHER MALE GENITAL | 0 | 0.02 | 0.0 | 0 | 0.02 | 0.0 | 0 | 0.0 | 0.0 |
| KIDNEY AND URETER | 2 | 0.37 | 5.36 | 0 | 0.14 | 0.0 | 2 | 0.23 | 8.70* |
| BLADDER | 3 | 0.81 | 3.68 | 1 | 0.43 | 2.35 | 2 | 0.39 | 5.15 |
| MELANOMA OF SKIN | 0 | 0.23 | 0.0 | 0 | 0.05 | 0.0 | 0 | 0.18 | 0.0 |
| EYE | 0 | 0.04 | 0.0 | 0 | 0.01 | 0.0 | 0 | 0.03 | 0.0 |
| NERVOUS SYSTEM | 0 | 0.29 | 0.0 | 0 | 0.08 | 0.0 | 0 | 0.22 | 0.0 |
| THYROID | 1 | 0.19 | 5.27 | 0 | 0.02 | 0.0 | 1 | 0.17 | 5.91 |
| BONE | 0 | 0.06 | 0.0 | 0 | 0.02 | 0.0 | 0 | 0.04 | 0.0 |
| SOFT TISSUE | 0 | 0.18 | 0.0 | 0 | 0.05 | 0.0 | 0 | 0.13 | 0.0 |
| LYMPHOMAS & MYELOMA | 3 | 0.67 | 4.46 | 2 | 0.19 | 10.52* | 1 | 0.48 | 2.07 |
| LEUKEMIAS | 2 | 0.54 | 3.68 | 0 | 0.18 | 0.0 | 2 | 0.36 | 5.52 |
| OTHER SITES | 4 | 1.15 | 3.47 | 0 | 0.33 | 0.0 | 4 | 0.82 | 4.89* |
| TOTAL | 41 | 23.06 | 1.78** | 4 | 6.02 | 0.66 | 37 | 17.04 | 2.17** |

Table 122. Subsequent primary sites with excesses

FIRST PRIMARY SITE - THYROID

| | TOTAL | | | YEARS < 1 | | | YEARS 1-5 | | | YEARS > 5 | | |
|---|---|---|---|---|---|---|---|---|---|---|---|---|
| | NUMBER OF PERSONS= 863<br>PERSON-YRS OF<br>OBSERVATION= 4428.2 | | | NUMBER OF PERSONS= 863<br>PERSON-YRS OF<br>OBSERVATION= 719.7 | | | NUMBER OF PERSONS= 637<br>PERSON-YRS OF<br>OBSERVATION= 1857.5 | | | NUMBER OF PERSONS= 329<br>PERSON-YRS OF<br>OBSERVATION= 1851.1 | | |
| SUBSEQUENT PRIMARY SITES | OBS | EXP | OBS/EXP | OBS | EXP | OBS/EXP | OBS | EXP | OBS/EXP | OBS | EXP | OBS/EXP |
| LIP | 1 | 0.11 | 9.21 | 0 | 0.02 | 0.0 | 1 | 0.05 | 20.97 | 0 | 0.04 | 0.0 |
| RECTUM | 5 | 1.32 | 3.78* | 0 | 0.23 | 0.0 | 4 | 0.52 | 7.62** | 1 | 0.57 | 1.76 |
| LARYNX | 2 | 0.20 | 10.14* | 1 | 0.03 | 29.03 | 0 | 0.08 | 0.0 | 1 | 0.08 | 12.32 |
| KIDNEY AND URETER | 2 | 0.37 | 5.36 | 1 | 0.06 | 16.26 | 0 | 0.15 | 0.0 | 1 | 0.17 | 6.03 |
| LYMPHOMAS & MYELOMA | 3 | 0.67 | 4.46 | 1 | 0.11 | 9.48 | 0 | 0.26 | 0.0 | 2 | 0.30 | 6.61 |
| LEUKEMIAS | 2 | 0.54 | 3.68 | 0 | 0.09 | 0.0 | 2 | 0.21 | 9.34* | 0 | 0.24 | 0.0 |
| OTHER SITES | 4 | 1.15 | 3.47 | 0 | 0.20 | 0.0 | 1 | 0.45 | 2.23 | 3 | 0.51 | 5.91* |

Table 123. Histologic confirmation of multiple primary malignancies

FIRST PRIMARY SITE - THYROID

| Subsequent primary site | Both tumor microscopically confirmed | | Only 1st tumor microscopically confirmed | | Only 2nd tumor microscopically confirmed | | Neither tumor microscopically confirmed | |
|---|---|---|---|---|---|---|---|---|
| | No. | % | No. | % | No. | % | No. | % |
| LIP | 1 | 100.0 | 0 | 0.0 | 0 | 0.0 | 0 | 0.0 |
| RECTUM | 4 | 80.0 | 1 | 20.0 | 0 | 0.0 | 0 | 0.0 |
| LARYNX | 1 | 50.0 | 1 | 50.0 | 0 | 0.0 | 0 | 0.0 |
| KIDNEY AND URETER | 2 | 100.0 | 0 | 0.0 | 0 | 0.0 | 0 | 0.0 |
| LYMPHOMAS & MYELOMA | 2 | 66.7 | 1 | 33.3 | 0 | 0.0 | 0 | 0.0 |
| LEUKEMIAS | 2 | 100.0 | 0 | 0.0 | 0 | 0.0 | 0 | 0.0 |
| OTHER SITES | 4 | 100.0 | 0 | 0.0 | 0 | 0.0 | 0 | 0.0 |

Table 124. Subsequent multiple primary malignancies in patients with an index malignant tumor of bone

FIRST PRIMARY SITE - BONE

| SUBSEQUENT PRIMARY SITES | TOTAL<br>NUMBER OF PERSONS= 511<br>PERSON-YRS OF OBSERVATION = 1864.3<br>OBS | <br><br><br>EXP | <br><br><br>OBS/EXP | MALES<br>NUMBER OF PERSONS= 288<br>PERSON-YRS OF OBSERVATION = 1007.7<br>OBS | <br><br><br>EXP | <br><br><br>OBS/EXP | FEMALES<br>NUMBER OF PERSONS= 223<br>PERSON-YRS OF OBSERVATION = 856.7<br>OBS | <br><br><br>EXP | <br><br><br>OBS/EXP |
|---|---|---|---|---|---|---|---|---|---|
| LIP | 0 | 0.09 | 0.0 | 0 | 0.08 | 0.0 | 0 | 0.00 | 0.0 |
| TONGUE | 0 | 0.07 | 0.0 | 0 | 0.07 | 0.0 | 0 | 0.01 | 0.0 |
| SALIVARY GLAND | 0 | 0.03 | 0.0 | 0 | 0.02 | 0.0 | 0 | 0.01 | 0.0 |
| MOUTH | 0 | 0.10 | 0.0 | 0 | 0.08 | 0.0 | 0 | 0.01 | 0.0 |
| PHARYNX | 0 | 0.10 | 0.0 | 0 | 0.09 | 0.0 | 0 | 0.01 | 0.0 |
| ESOPHAGUS | 0 | 0.17 | 0.0 | 0 | 0.15 | 0.0 | 0 | 0.02 | 0.0 |
| STOMACH | 1 | 0.69 | 1.45 | 1 | 0.51 | 1.95 | 0 | 0.18 | 0.0 |
| SMALL INTESTINE | 0 | 0.03 | 0.0 | 0 | 0.02 | 0.0 | 0 | 0.01 | 0.0 |
| COLON | 0 | 0.97 | 0.0 | 0 | 0.57 | 0.0 | 0 | 0.41 | 0.0 |
| RECTUM | 1 | 0.57 | 1.75 | 1 | 0.39 | 2.58 | 0 | 0.18 | 0.0 |
| LIVER & BILIARY PASS | 0 | 0.19 | 0.0 | 0 | 0.11 | 0.0 | 0 | 0.08 | 0.0 |
| PANCREAS | 0 | 0.27 | 0.0 | 0 | 0.19 | 0.0 | 0 | 0.08 | 0.0 |
| NOSE AND SINUSES | 0 | 0.02 | 0.0 | 0 | 0.01 | 0.0 | 0 | 0.00 | 0.0 |
| LARYNX | 1 | 0.12 | 8.27 | 0 | 0.11 | 0.0 | 1 | 0.01 | 137.88* |
| LUNG AND BRONCHUS | 0 | 0.69 | 0.0 | 0 | 0.61 | 0.0 | 0 | 0.08 | 0.0 |
| OTHER RESP | 0 | 0.01 | 0.0 | 0 | 0.01 | 0.0 | 0 | 0.00 | 0.0 |
| BREAST | 0 | 0.82 | 0.0 | 0 | 0.01 | 0.0 | 0 | 0.81 | 0.0 |
| CERVIX UTERI | 0 | 0.30 | 0.0 | 0 | 0.0 | 0.0 | 0 | 0.30 | 0.0 |
| CORPUS UTERI | 0 | 0.17 | 0.0 | 0 | 0.0 | 0.0 | 0 | 0.17 | 0.0 |
| UTERUS,UNSPEC | 1 | 0.09 | 10.90 | 0 | 0.0 | 0.0 | 1 | 0.09 | 10.90 |
| OVARY | 0 | 0.17 | 0.0 | 0 | 0.0 | 0.0 | 0 | 0.17 | 0.0 |
| OTHER FEMALE GENITAL | 0 | 0.03 | 0.0 | 0 | 0.0 | 0.0 | 0 | 0.03 | 0.0 |
| PROSTATE | 3 | 0.88 | 3.39 | 3 | 0.88 | 3.39 | 0 | 0.0 | 0.0 |
| TESTIS | 0 | 0.03 | 0.0 | 0 | 0.03 | 0.0 | 0 | 0.0 | 0.0 |
| OTHER MALE GENITAL | 0 | 0.02 | 0.0 | 0 | 0.02 | 0.0 | 0 | 0.0 | 0.0 |
| KIDNEY AND URETER | 0 | 0.16 | 0.0 | 0 | 0.11 | 0.0 | 0 | 0.05 | 0.0 |
| BLADDER | 0 | 0.44 | 0.0 | 0 | 0.36 | 0.0 | 0 | 0.08 | 0.0 |
| MELANOMA OF SKIN | 0 | 0.07 | 0.0 | 0 | 0.04 | 0.0 | 0 | 0.03 | 0.0 |
| EYE | 0 | 0.02 | 0.0 | 0 | 0.01 | 0.0 | 0 | 0.01 | 0.0 |
| NERVOUS SYSTEM | 0 | 0.10 | 0.0 | 0 | 0.06 | 0.0 | 0 | 0.04 | 0.0 |
| THYROID | 0 | 0.05 | 0.0 | 0 | 0.02 | 0.0 | 0 | 0.03 | 0.0 |
| BONE | 0 | 0.03 | 0.0 | 0 | 0.02 | 0.0 | 0 | 0.01 | 0.0 |
| SOFT TISSUE | 1 | 0.06 | 16.89 | 0 | 0.04 | 0.0 | 1 | 0.02 | 41.43* |
| LYMPHOMAS & MYELOMA | 0 | 0.25 | 0.0 | 0 | 0.16 | 0.0 | 0 | 0.09 | 0.0 |
| LEUKEMIAS | 0 | 0.23 | 0.0 | 0 | 0.16 | 0.0 | 0 | 0.07 | 0.0 |
| OTHER SITES | 3 | 0.43 | 7.06* | 2 | 0.26 | 7.62 | 1 | 0.16 | 6.15 |
| TOTAL | 11 | 8.45 | 1.30 | 7 | 5.18 | 1.35 | 4 | 3.27 | 1.22 |

Table 125. Subsequent primary sites with excesses

FIRST PRIMARY SITE - BONE

| SUBSEQUENT PRIMARY SITES | TOTAL | | | YEARS < 1 | | | YEARS 1-5 | | | YEARS > 5 | | |
|---|---|---|---|---|---|---|---|---|---|---|---|---|
| | NUMBER OF PERSONS= 511 PERSON-YRS OF OBSERVATION= 1864.3 | | | NUMBER OF PERSONS= 511 PERSON-YRS OF OBSERVATION= 385.7 | | | NUMBER OF PERSONS= 282 PERSON-YRS OF OBSERVATION= 679.7 | | | NUMBER OF PERSONS= 110 PERSON-YRS OF OBSERVATION= 798.8 | | |
| | OBS | EXP | OBS/EXP | OBS | EXP | OBS/EXP | OBS | EXP | OBS/EXP | OBS | EXP | OBS/EXP |
| LARYNX | 1 | 0.12 | 8.27 | 1 | 0.02 | 41.15* | 0 | 0.04 | 0.0 | 0 | 0.06 | 0.0 |
| PROSTATE | 3 | 0.88 | 3.39 | 2 | 0.14 | 14.25* | 1 | 0.27 | 3.72 | 0 | 0.48 | 0.0 |
| SOFT TISSUE | 1 | 0.06 | 16.89 | 0 | 0.01 | 0.0 | 1 | 0.02 | 53.04* | 0 | 0.03 | 0.0 |
| OTHER SITES | 3 | 0.43 | 7.06* | 0 | 0.08 | 0.0 | 2 | 0.13 | 15.63* | 1 | 0.22 | 4.61 |

Table 126. Histologic confirmation of multiple primary malignancies

FIRST PRIMARY SITE - BONE

| Subsequent primary site | Both tumors microscopically confirmed | | Only 1st tumor microscopically confirmed | | Only 2nd tumor microscopically confirmed | | Neither tumor microscopically confirmed | |
|---|---|---|---|---|---|---|---|---|
| | No. | % | No. | % | No. | % | No. | % |
| LARYNX | 0 | 0.0 | 0 | 0.0 | 0 | 0.0 | 1 | 100.0 |
| PROSTATE | 2 | 66.7 | 0 | 0.0 | 1 | 33.3 | 0 | 0.0 |
| SOFT TISSUE | 1 | 100.0 | 0 | 0.0 | 0 | 0.0 | 0 | 0.0 |
| OTHER SITES | 2 | 66.7 | 1 | 33.3 | 0 | 0.0 | 0 | 0.0 |

Table 127. Subsequent multiple primary malignancies in patients with an index malignant tumor of soft tissue

FIRST PRIMARY SITE - SOFT TISSUE

| SUBSEQUENT PRIMARY SITES | TOTAL | | | MALES | | | FEMALES | | |
|---|---|---|---|---|---|---|---|---|---|
| | NUMBER OF PERSONS= 1119 PERSON-YRS OF OBSERVATION = 6114.2 | | | NUMBER OF PERSONS= 598 PERSON-YRS OF OBSERVATION = 3032.5 | | | NUMBER OF PERSONS= 521 PERSON-YRS OF OBSERVATION = 3081.7 | | |
| | OBS | EXP | OBS/EXP | OBS | EXP | OBS/EXP | OBS | EXP | OBS/EXP |
| LIP | 0 | 0.40 | 0.0 | 0 | 0.38 | 0.0 | 0 | 0.02 | 0.0 |
| TONGUE | 1 | 0.36 | 2.76 | 1 | 0.32 | 3.16 | 0 | 0.05 | 0.0 |
| SALIVARY GLAND | 0 | 0.12 | 0.0 | 0 | 0.08 | 0.0 | 0 | 0.05 | 0.0 |
| MOUTH | 0 | 0.47 | 0.0 | 0 | 0.39 | 0.0 | 0 | 0.08 | 0.0 |
| PHARYNX | 0 | 0.46 | 0.0 | 0 | 0.39 | 0.0 | 0 | 0.07 | 0.0 |
| ESOPHAGUS | 1 | 0.79 | 1.27 | 1 | 0.70 | 1.43 | 0 | 0.09 | 0.0 |
| STOMACH | 4 | 3.41 | 1.17 | 2 | 2.38 | 0.84 | 2 | 1.03 | 1.94 |
| SMALL INTESTINE | 0 | 0.14 | 0.0 | 0 | 0.08 | 0.0 | 0 | 0.06 | 0.0 |
| COLON | 13 | 5.11 | 2.54** | 6 | 2.75 | 2.18 | 7 | 2.36 | 2.97* |
| RECTUM | 5 | 2.82 | 1.77 | 3 | 1.80 | 1.66 | 2 | 1.02 | 1.97 |
| LIVER & BILIARY PASS | 1 | 0.99 | 1.01 | 0 | 0.51 | 0.0 | 1 | 0.48 | 2.09 |
| PANCREAS | 2 | 1.41 | 1.42 | 1 | 0.90 | 1.11 | 1 | 0.50 | 1.98 |
| NOSE AND SINUSES | 0 | 0.09 | 0.0 | 0 | 0.06 | 0.0 | 0 | 0.03 | 0.0 |
| LARYNX | 0 | 0.59 | 0.0 | 0 | 0.55 | 0.0 | 0 | 0.04 | 0.0 |
| LUNG AND BRONCHUS | 2 | 3.47 | 0.58 | 2 | 3.04 | 0.66 | 0 | 0.44 | 0.0 |
| OTHER RESP | 0 | 0.07 | 0.0 | 0 | 0.05 | 0.0 | 0 | 0.02 | 0.0 |
| BREAST | 2 | 4.37 | 0.46 | 0 | 0.06 | 0.0 | 2 | 4.31 | 0.46 |
| CERVIX UTERI | 1 | 1.31 | 0.77 | 0 | 0.0 | 0.0 | 1 | 1.31 | 0.77 |
| CORPUS UTERI | 3 | 0.91 | 3.30 | 0 | 0.0 | 0.0 | 3 | 0.91 | 3.30 |
| UTERUS,UNSPEC | 0 | 0.46 | 0.0 | 0 | 0.0 | 0.0 | 0 | 0.46 | 0.0 |
| OVARY | 1 | 0.87 | 1.15 | 0 | 0.0 | 0.0 | 1 | 0.87 | 1.15 |
| OTHER FEMALE GENITAL | 0 | 0.17 | 0.0 | 0 | 0.0 | 0.0 | 0 | 0.17 | 0.0 |
| PROSTATE | 6 | 4.32 | 1.39 | 6 | 4.32 | 1.39 | 0 | 0.0 | 0.0 |
| TESTIS | 0 | 0.08 | 0.0 | 0 | 0.08 | 0.0 | 0 | 0.0 | 0.0 |
| OTHER MALE GENITAL | 0 | 0.09 | 0.0 | 0 | 0.09 | 0.0 | 0 | 0.0 | 0.0 |
| KIDNEY AND URETER | 0 | 0.79 | 0.0 | 0 | 0.54 | 0.0 | 0 | 0.25 | 0.0 |
| BLADDER | 5 | 2.21 | 2.26 | 3 | 1.75 | 1.72 | 2 | 0.47 | 4.30 |
| MELANOMA OF SKIN | 1 | 0.31 | 3.18 | 1 | 0.16 | 6.34 | 0 | 0.16 | 0.0 |
| EYE | 1 | 0.08 | 12.76 | 1 | 0.04 | 22.86 | 0 | 0.03 | 0.0 |
| NERVOUS SYSTEM | 1 | 0.43 | 2.34 | 0 | 0.23 | 0.0 | 1 | 0.20 | 5.12 |
| THYROID | 0 | 0.22 | 0.0 | 0 | 0.07 | 0.0 | 0 | 0.15 | 0.0 |
| BONE | 0 | 0.12 | 0.0 | 0 | 0.07 | 0.0 | 0 | 0.05 | 0.0 |
| SOFT TISSUE | 2 | 0.29 | 6.96 | 0 | 0.16 | 0.0 | 2 | 0.12 | 16.28* |
| LYMPHOMAS & MYELOMA | 0 | 1.15 | 0.0 | 0 | 0.68 | 0.0 | 0 | 0.48 | 0.0 |
| LEUKEMIAS | 1 | 1.15 | 0.87 | 1 | 0.74 | 1.36 | 0 | 0.41 | 0.0 |
| OTHER SITES | 1 | 2.23 | 0.45 | 1 | 1.28 | 0.78 | 0 | 0.95 | 0.0 |
| TOTAL | 54 | 42.25 | 1.28 | 29 | 24.64 | 1.18 | 25 | 17.61 | 1.42 |

Table 128. Subsequent primary sites with excesses

FIRST PRIMARY SITE - SOFT TISSUE

| | TOTAL | | | YEARS < 1 | | | YEARS 1-5 | | | YEARS > 5 | | |
|---|---|---|---|---|---|---|---|---|---|---|---|---|
| | NUMBER OF PERSONS= 1119<br>PERSON-YRS OF<br>OBSERVATION= 6114.2 | | | NUMBER OF PERSONS= 1119<br>PERSON-YRS OF<br>OBSERVATION= 941.7 | | | NUMBER OF PERSONS= 811<br>PERSON-YRS OF<br>OBSERVATION= 2309.0 | | | NUMBER OF PERSONS= 409<br>PERSON-YRS OF<br>OBSERVATION= 2863.4 | | |
| SUBSEQUENT PRIMARY SITES | OBS | EXP | OBS/EXP | OBS | EXP | OBS/EXP | OBS | EXP | OBS/EXP | OBS | EXP | OBS/EXP |
| COLON | 13 | 5.11 | 2.54** | 2 | 0.72 | 2.79 | 5 | 1.73 | 2.88 | 6 | 2.66 | 2.26 |
| PROSTATE | 6 | 4.32 | 1.39 | 3 | 0.60 | 4.98* | 0 | 1.37 | 0.0 | 3 | 2.35 | 1.28 |
| EYE | 1 | 0.08 | 12.76 | 1 | 0.01 | 91.02* | 0 | 0.03 | 0.0 | 0 | 0.04 | 0.0 |
| SOFT TISSUE | 2 | 0.29 | 6.96 | 0 | 0.04 | 0.0 | 1 | 0.10 | 10.07 | 1 | 0.15 | 6.87 |

Table 129. Histologic confirmation of multiple primary malignancies

FIRST PRIMARY SITE - SOFT TISSUE

| Subsequent primary site | Both tumors microscopically confirmed | | Only 1st tumor microscopically confirmed | | Only 2nd tumor microscopically confirmed | | Neither tumor microscopically confirmed | |
|---|---|---|---|---|---|---|---|---|
| | No. | % | No. | % | No. | % | No. | % |
| COLON | 11 | 84.6 | 2 | 15.4 | 0 | 0.0 | 0 | 0.0 |
| PROSTATE | 1 | 16.7 | 4 | 66.7 | 0 | 0.0 | 1 | 16.7 |
| EYE | 1 | 100.0 | 0 | 0.0 | 0 | 0.0 | 0 | 0.0 |
| SOFT TISSUE | 2 | 100.0 | 0 | 0.0 | 0 | 0.0 | 0 | 0.0 |

Table 130. Subsequent multiple primary malignancies in patients with an index malidnant tumor of other and unspecified sites

FIRST PRIMARY SITE - OTHER AND UNSPECIFIED SITES

| | TOTAL | | | MALES | | | FEMALES | | |
|---|---|---|---|---|---|---|---|---|---|
| | NUMBER OF PERSONS= 4825<br>PERSON-YRS OF<br>OBSERVATION = 4537.0 | | | NUMBER OF PERSONS= 2462<br>PERSON-YRS OF<br>OBSERVATION = 2201.0 | | | NUMBER OF PERSONS= 2363<br>PERSON-YRS OF<br>OBSERVATION = 2336.0 | | |
| SUBSEQUENT PRIMARY SITES | OBS | EXP | OBS/EXP | OBS | EXP | OBS/EXP | OBS | EXP | OBS/EXP |
| LIP | 1 | 0.39 | 2.59 | 1 | 0.36 | 2.77 | 0 | 0.02 | 0.0 |
| TONGUE | 1 | 0.34 | 2.96 | 1 | 0.29 | 3.46 | 0 | 0.05 | 0.0 |
| SALIVARY GLAND | 0 | 0.12 | 0.0 | 0 | 0.07 | 0.0 | 0 | 0.05 | 0.0 |
| MOUTH | 0 | 0.45 | 0.0 | 0 | 0.36 | 0.0 | 0 | 0.09 | 0.0 |
| PHARYNX | 0 | 0.44 | 0.0 | 0 | 0.37 | 0.0 | 0 | 0.07 | 0.0 |
| ESOPHAGUS | 1 | 0.76 | 1.32 | 1 | 0.64 | 1.55 | 0 | 0.11 | 0.0 |
| STOMACH | 2 | 3.54 | 0.57 | 2 | 2.23 | 0.90 | 0 | 1.30 | 0.0 |
| SMALL INTESTINE | 0 | 0.15 | 0.0 | 0 | 0.08 | 0.0 | 0 | 0.07 | 0.0 |
| COLON | 4 | 5.31 | 0.75 | 2 | 2.57 | 0.78 | 2 | 2.75 | 0.73 |
| RECTUM | 1 | 2.81 | 0.36 | 1 | 1.66 | 0.60 | 0 | 1.15 | 0.0 |
| LIVER & BILIARY PASS | 0 | 1.08 | 0.0 | 0 | 0.49 | 0.0 | 0 | 0.60 | 0.0 |
| PANCREAS | 1 | 1.44 | 0.69 | 0 | 0.85 | 0.0 | 1 | 0.59 | 1.69 |
| NOSE AND SINUSES | 0 | 0.08 | 0.0 | 0 | 0.05 | 0.0 | 0 | 0.03 | 0.0 |
| LARYNX | 0 | 0.55 | 0.0 | 0 | 0.51 | 0.0 | 0 | 0.03 | 0.0 |
| LUNG AND BRONCHUS | 4 | 3.32 | 1.20 | 4 | 2.85 | 1.40 | 0 | 0.48 | 0.0 |
| OTHER RESP | 0 | 0.06 | 0.0 | 0 | 0.05 | 0.0 | 0 | 0.01 | 0.0 |
| BREAST | 3 | 4.40 | 0.68 | 0 | 0.06 | 0.0 | 3 | 4.35 | 0.69 |
| CERVIX UTERI | 2 | 1.05 | 1.91 | 0 | 0.0 | 0.0 | 2 | 1.05 | 1.91 |
| CORPUS UTERI | 0 | 0.89 | 0.0 | 0 | 0.0 | 0.0 | 0 | 0.89 | 0.0 |
| UTERUS, UNSPEC | 0 | 0.53 | 0.0 | 0 | 0.0 | 0.0 | 0 | 0.53 | 0.0 |
| OVARY | 0 | 0.83 | 0.0 | 0 | 0.0 | 0.0 | 0 | 0.83 | 0.0 |
| OTHER FEMALE GENITAL | 0 | 0.20 | 0.0 | 0 | 0.0 | 0.0 | 0 | 0.20 | 0.0 |
| PROSTATE | 4 | 4.00 | 1.00 | 4 | 4.00 | 1.00 | 0 | 0.0 | 0.0 |
| TESTIS | 0 | 0.05 | 0.0 | 0 | 0.05 | 0.0 | 0 | 0.0 | 0.0 |
| OTHER MALE GENITAL | 0 | 0.08 | 0.0 | 0 | 0.08 | 0.0 | 0 | 0.0 | 0.0 |
| KIDNEY AND URETER | 3 | 0.77 | 3.91 | 3 | 0.49 | 6.12* | 0 | 0.28 | 0.0 |
| BLADDER | 1 | 2.16 | 0.46 | 0 | 1.60 | 0.0 | 1 | 0.56 | 1.78 |
| MELANOMA OF SKIN | 0 | 0.27 | 0.0 | 0 | 0.13 | 0.0 | 0 | 0.14 | 0.0 |
| EYE | 0 | 0.08 | 0.0 | 0 | 0.04 | 0.0 | 0 | 0.04 | 0.0 |
| NERVOUS SYSTEM | 0 | 0.37 | 0.0 | 0 | 0.20 | 0.0 | 0 | 0.17 | 0.0 |
| THYROID | 2 | 0.20 | 9.97* | 2 | 0.06 | 32.70** | 0 | 0.14 | 0.0 |
| BONE | 0 | 0.11 | 0.0 | 0 | 0.06 | 0.0 | 0 | 0.05 | 0.0 |
| SOFT TISSUE | 0 | 0.25 | 0.0 | 0 | 0.14 | 0.0 | 0 | 0.11 | 0.0 |
| LYMPHOMAS & MYELOMA | 0 | 1.08 | 0.0 | 0 | 0.60 | 0.0 | 0 | 0.47 | 0.0 |
| LEUKEMIAS | 4 | 1.09 | 3.67* | 2 | 0.66 | 3.04 | 2 | 0.43 | 4.62 |
| OTHER SITES | 1 | 2.33 | 0.43 | 1 | 1.21 | 0.83 | 0 | 1.12 | 0.0 |
| TOTAL | 35 | 41.58 | 0.84 | 24 | 22.80 | 1.05 | 11 | 18.78 | 0.59 |

Table 131. Subsequent primary sites with excesses

FIRST PRIMARY SITE - OTHER AND UNSPECIFIED SITES

| SUBSEQUENT PRIMARY SITES | TOTAL | | | YEARS < 1 | | | YEARS 1-5 | | | YEARS > 5 | | |
|---|---|---|---|---|---|---|---|---|---|---|---|---|
| | NUMBER OF PERSONS= 4825<br>PERSON-YRS OF OBSERVATION= 4537.0 | | | NUMBER OF PERSONS= 4825<br>PERSON-YRS OF OBSERVATION= 2035.2 | | | NUMBER OF PERSONS= 897<br>PERSON-YRS OF OBSERVATION= 1533.3 | | | NUMBER OF PERSONS= 182<br>PERSON-YRS OF OBSERVATION= 967.9 | | |
| | OBS | EXP | OBS/EXP | OBS | EXP | OBS/EXP | OBS | EXP | OBS/EXP | OBS | EXP | OBS/EXP |
| KIDNEY AND URETER | 3 | 0.77 | 3.91 | 1 | 0.35 | 2.84 | 1 | 0.24 | 4.10 | 1 | 0.17 | 5.83 |
| THYROID | 2 | 0.20 | 9.97* | 1 | 0.09 | 11.34 | 1 | 0.07 | 15.27 | 0 | 0.05 | 0.0 |
| LEUKEMIAS | 4 | 1.09 | 3.67* | 3 | 0.49 | 6.07* | 1 | 0.35 | 2.89 | 0 | 0.25 | 0.0 |

Table 132. Histologic confirmation of multiple primary malignancies

FIRST PRIMARY SITE - OTHER AND UNSPECIFIED SITES

| Subsequent primary site | Both tumors microscopically confirmed | | Only 1st tumor microscopically confirmed | | Only 2nd tumor microscopically confirmed | | Neither tumor microscopically confirmed | |
|---|---|---|---|---|---|---|---|---|
| | No. | % | No. | % | No. | % | No. | % |
| KIDNEY AND URETER | 2 | 66.7 | 0 | 0.0 | 1 | 33.3 | 0 | 0.0 |
| THYROID | 2 | 100.0 | 0 | 0.0 | 0 | 0.0 | 0 | 0.0 |
| LEUKEMIAS | 2 | 50.0 | 0 | 0.0 | 2 | 50.0 | 0 | 0.0 |

Table 133. Summary of site-group pairs with an excess of observed-over-expected subsequent primary malignancies: index tumors of remaining and ill-defined sites

I. Possibly artifact

Malignant melanoma (skin) ----------------➤ Salivary gland
Malignant melanoma (skin) ----------------➤ Esophagus
Malignant melanoma (skin) ----------------➤ Rectum
Malignant melanoma (skin) ----------------➤ Other/unspecified sites
Nervous system ---------------------------➤ Prostate
Nervous system ---------------------------➤ Kidney/ureter
Nervous system ---------------------------➤ Thyroid
Nervous system ---------------------------➤ Lymphoma/myeloma
Thyroid ----------------------------------➤ Lip
Thyroid ----------------------------------➤ Rectum
Thyroid ----------------------------------➤ Larynx
Thyroid ----------------------------------➤ Kidney/ureter
Thyroid ----------------------------------➤ Lymphoma/myeloma
Thyroid ➤---------------------------------➤ Other/unspecified sites
Bone -------------------------------------➤ Larynx
Bone -------------------------------------➤ Prostate
Bone -------------------------------------➤ Soft tissue
Bone -------------------------------------➤ Other/unspecified sites
Soft tissue ------------------------------➤ Prostate
Soft tissue ------------------------------➤ Eye
Other/unspecified sites ------------------➤ Kidney/ureter
Other/unspecified sites ------------------➤ Leukemia

II. Possibly real

A. In organs within the same system

1. Same or paired organs

Malignant melanoma (skin) ➤---------------➤ Malignant melanoma (skin)
Eye ➤-------------------------------------➤ Eye

2. Other

Soft tissue ➤-----------------------------➤ Soft tissue

B. In organs related structurally or functionally

None

C. In organs apparently unrelated structurally or functionally

Eye --------------------------------------➤ Bone
Nervous system ---------------------------➤ Breast
Thyroid ----------------------------------➤ Leukemia
Soft tissue ------------------------------➤ Colon
Malignant melanoma (skin) ----------------➤ Breast

Table 134. Common metastatic sites for primary malignant tumors of remaining sites (HOLLAND and FREI, 1973; WILLIS, 1973; RUBIN, 1974)

| Anatomic location of the primary malignant tumor | Common metastatic sites |
|---|---|
| Malignant melanoma (skin) | Lymph nodes; skin; lung; liver; bone; gastrointestinal sites; brain; kidney; heart; adrenals; spleen |
| Eye | Central nervous system (in retinoblastoma) |
| Brain | Other sites in the central nervous system |
| Thyroid | Bone; mediastinal and cervical lymph nodes; lung |
| Bone | Spine; skull; pelvis |
| Soft-tissue sarcomas | Regional lymph nodes; lung |

# Chapter 13

# Summary, Applications of these Data, and Perspectives for the Future

Summary. Results for non-simultaneously diagnosed malignant tumors from Connecticut indicate that individuals with one malignant neoplasm have 1.29 times the risk of developing a new independent primary tumor when compared to individuals who never had cancer ($P < 0.01$). However, the increased risk of multiple primary tumors is highly selective on a site-specific basis. Table 135 presents Connecticut Registry data indicating the risk of a subsequent primary malignancy by anatomic site of the later primary in patients with a first primary cancer. Tables 136 and 137 present tabulations for anatomic sites with statistically significant excesses and deficiencies, with an analysis by time interval between the two malignancies. Finally, Table 138 presents figures showing histologic confirmation for site-group pairs with significant excesses of observed-over-expected later primary malignant neoplasms.

The reader should bear in mind that just as the risk of subsequent primaries varies with the anatomic site of the subsequent primary (Table 135), the risk is also highly dependent upon the anatomic site of the first primary cancer (Chapters 6-12).

Application of These Data. Studies of multiple primary malignancies derived from the experience of a population-based tumor registry are of immediate value in cancer control programs. Findings of such studies highlight particular organs or tissues most likely to develop a second primary cancer, and are useful to the clinician concerned with detecting the second malignancy at the earliest possible stage.

The tabulations in this monograph better define the risk in the cancer patient of subsequent primary malignancies in terms of sex, tumor site, and time interval between the tumors. These data also help clarify the carcinogenic potential of various treatment modalities currently employed in the care of the cancer patient. When applied to questions of etiology, such studies provide corroboration for other epidemiologic investigations into the pathogenesis and causes of cancer. The results serve to complement the findings of genetic studies. Discovering hitherto unsuspected relationships between tumors may permit one to apply what is currently known about one tumor to understand the etiology of an associated neoplasm. Finally, reports of multiple primary cancers should assist in the identification of particular segments of the population for further study to elucidate the factors and mechanisms involved in oncogenesis.

Perspectives for the Future. The findings of this study of multiple primary neoplasms do not provide definitive answers, but rather are useful in formulating and testing hypotheses. One must be cautious to distinguish: 1) real from arctifactual relationships and 2) biologic from statistical significance. Other studies are needed to corroborate and evaluate the findings concerning multiple primaries. Detailed reviews of case histories and pathologic specimens should be undertaken to test the relationships suggested. As we are able to follow larger population groups of cancer patients over longer periods, it will be possible to define the risk of subsequent primary cancer with more precision, not only in terms of sex, tumor site, and time interval between tumors as demonstrated in this monograph, but also in terms of the histologic type of the associated neoplasms. Such an analysis requires nearly complete microscopic confirmation of both the first and subsequent primary tumor.

It will also be useful to abstract and collect more detailed information on therapeutic regimens to evaluate better the carcinogenic potential of these various treatment modalities.

Finally, one should carefully examine results for patients at low risk for multiple primary cancer. Provided the deficits in observed-over-expected subsequent primary malignancies discovered in the Connecticut data are confirmed by other investigations, this information may be fruitful in detecting the mechanism involved in the reduction of risk. Such findings would be most applicable to efforts aimed at the primary prevention of malignant neoplasms.

Table 135. Subsequent multiple primary malignancies in patients with an index malignant tumor of any site (excluding non-melanotic skin cancer)

FIRST PRIMARY SITE - ALL SITES

| SUBSEQUENT PRIMARY SITES | TOTAL | | | MALES | | | FEMALES | | |
|---|---|---|---|---|---|---|---|---|---|
| | NUMBER OF PERSONS= 121460 PERSON-YRS OF OBSERVATION = 419382.9 | | | NUMBER OF PERSONS= 56404 PERSON-YRS OF OBSERVATION = 146875.4 | | | NUMBER OF PERSONS= 65056 PERSON-YRS OF OBSERVATION = 272507.4 | | |
| | OBS | EXP | OBS/EXP | OBS | EXP | OBS/EXP | OBS | EXP | OBS/EXP |
| LIP | 43 | 30.46 | 1.41* | 38 | 27.87 | 1.36 | 5 | 2.59 | 1.93 |
| TONGUE | 71 | 28.08 | 2.53** | 66 | 22.52 | 2.93** | 5 | 5.56 | 0.90 |
| SALIVARY GLAND | 16 | 11.02 | 1.45 | 10 | 5.30 | 1.89 | 6 | 5.72 | 1.05 |
| MOUTH | 79 | 37.64 | 2.10** | 56 | 28.47 | 1.97** | 23 | 9.18 | 2.51** |
| PHARYNX | 65 | 36.02 | 1.80** | 47 | 28.20 | 1.67** | 18 | 7.82 | 2.30** |
| ESOPHAGUS | 75 | 62.62 | 1.20 | 59 | 50.99 | 1.16 | 16 | 11.63 | 1.38 |
| STOMACH | 227 | 305.98 | 0.74** | 124 | 175.42 | 0.71** | 103 | 130.56 | 0.79* |
| SMALL INTESTINE | 23 | 13.47 | 1.71* | 11 | 5.88 | 1.87 | 12 | 7.60 | 1.58 |
| COLON | 655 | 496.44 | 1.32** | 268 | 208.70 | 1.28** | 387 | 287.74 | 1.34** |
| RECTUM | 304 | 256.46 | 1.19** | 141 | 132.66 | 1.06 | 163 | 123.80 | 1.32** |
| LIVER & BILIARY PASS | 85 | 98.79 | 0.86 | 34 | 38.47 | 0.88 | 51 | 60.32 | 0.85 |
| PANCREAS | 116 | 130.56 | 0.89 | 67 | 68.68 | 0.98 | 49 | 61.88 | 0.79 |
| NOSE AND SINUSES | 11 | 7.38 | 1.49 | 4 | 4.07 | 0.98 | 7 | 3.31 | 2.11 |
| LARYNX | 51 | 43.98 | 1.16 | 43 | 39.86 | 1.08 | 8 | 4.12 | 1.94 |
| LUNG AND BRONCHUS | 331 | 278.00 | 1.19** | 253 | 226.09 | 1.12 | 78 | 51.91 | 1.50** |
| OTHER RESP | 9 | 5.04 | 1.78 | 5 | 3.47 | 1,44 | 4 | 1.58 | 2.54 |
| BREAST | 944 | 492.64 | 1.92** | 7 | 4.38 | 1.60 | 937 | 488.27 | 1.92** |
| CERVIX UTERI | 112 | 127.85 | 0.88 | 0 | 0.0 | 0.0 | 112 | 127.85 | 0.88 |
| CORPUS UTERI | 157 | 104.99 | 1.50** | 0 | 0.0 | 0.0 | 157 | 104.99 | 1.50** |
| UTERUS,UNSPEC | 49 | 56.66 | 0.86 | 0 | 0.0 | 0.0 | 49 | 56.66 | 0.86 |
| OVARY | 172 | 97.19 | 1.77** | 0 | 0.0 | 0.0 | 172 | 97.19 | 1.77** |
| OTHER FEMALE GENITAL | 39 | 20.82 | 1.87** | 0 | 0.0 | 0.0 | 39 | 20.82 | 1.87** |
| PROSTATE | 459 | 342.80 | 1.34** | 459 | 342.80 | 1.34** | 0 | 0.0 | 0.0 |
| TESTIS | 12 | 3.59 | 3.34** | 12 | 3.59 | 3.34** | 0 | 0.0 | 0.0 |
| OTHER MALE GENITAL | 5 | 6.55 | 0.76 | 5 | 6.55 | 0.76 | 0 | 0.0 | 0.0 |
| KIDNEY AND URETER | 119 | 69.10 | 1.72** | 81 | 39.01 | 2.08** | 38 | 30.09 | 1.26 |
| BLADDER | 239 | 189.25 | 1.26** | 138 | 131.89 | 1.05 | 101 | 57.37 | 1.76** |
| MELANOMA OF SKIN | 45 | 26.01 | 1.73** | 25 | 9.92 | 2.52** | 20 | 16.09 | 1.24 |
| EYE | 15 | 7.15 | 2.10* | 4 | 3.12 | 1.28 | 11 | 4.03 | 2.73** |
| NERVOUS SYSTEM | 21 | 33.90 | 0.62* | 8 | 13.09 | 0.61 | 13 | 20.82 | 0.62 |
| THYROID | 30 | 20.32 | 1.48 | 13 | 4.79 | 2.72** | 17 | 15.54 | 1.09 |
| BONE | 11 | 10.06 | 1.09 | 5 | 4.41 | 1.13 | 6 | 5.65 | 1.06 |
| SOFT TISSUE | 48 | 24.08 | 1.99** | 17 | 11.38 | 1.49 | 31 | 12.70 | 2.44** |
| LYMPHOMAS & MYELOMA | 98 | 99.95 | 0.98 | 47 | 46.55 | 1.01 | 51 | 53.40 | 0.96 |
| LEUKEMIAS | 118 | 100.85 | 1.17 | 77 | 53.52 | 1.44** | 41 | 47.33 | 0.87 |
| OTHER SITES | 168 | 211.34 | 0.79** | 84 | 96.90 | 0.87 | 84 | 114.45 | 0.73** |
| TOTAL | 5022 | 3887.05 | 1.29** | 2208 | 1838.52 | 1.20** | 2814 | 2048.53 | 1.37** |

Table 136. Subsequent primary sites with excesses (excluding non-melanotic skin cancer)

FIRST PRIMARY - ALL SITES (excluding non-melanotic skin cancer)

| | TOTAL | | | YEARS < 1 | | | YEARS 1-5 | | | YEARS > 5 | | |
|---|---|---|---|---|---|---|---|---|---|---|---|---|
| | NUMBER OF PERSONS=121460 PERSON-YRS OF OBSERVATION= 419382.9 | | | NUMBER OF PERSONS=121460 PERSON-YRS OF OBSERVATION= 88408.9 | | | NUMBER OF PERSONS= 69292 PERSON-YRS OF OBSERVATION= 170850.1 | | | NUMBER OF PERSONS= 27551 PERSON-YRS OF OBSERVATION= 160123.9 | | |
| SUBSEQUENT PRIMARY SITES | OBS | EXP | OBS/EXP | OBS | EXP | OBS/EXP | OBS | EXP | OBS/EXP | OBS | EXP | OBS/EXP |
| LIP | 43 | 30.46 | 1.41* | 11 | 7.31 | 1.50 | 22 | 12.56 | 1.75* | 10 | 10.59 | 0.94 |
| TONGUE | 71 | 28.08 | 2.53** | 14 | 6.43 | 2.18* | 34 | 11.47 | 2.96** | 23 | 10.18 | 2.26** |
| MOUTH | 79 | 37.64 | 2.10** | 12 | 8.40 | 1.43 | 35 | 15.18 | 2.31** | 32 | 14.07 | 2.27** |
| PHARYNX | 65 | 36.02 | 1.80** | 16 | 8.14 | 1.97* | 28 | 14.67 | 1.91** | 21 | 13.20 | 1.59 |
| ESOPHAGUS | 75 | 62.62 | 1.20 | 14 | 14.49 | 0.97 | 38 | 25.74 | 1.48* | 23 | 22.39 | 1.03 |
| SMALL INTESTINE | 23 | 13.47 | 1.71* | 6 | 2.69 | 2.23 | 10 | 5.24 | 1.91 | 7 | 5.55 | 1.26 |
| COLON | 655 | 496.44 | 1.32** | 110 | 95.60 | 1.15 | 234 | 189.77 | 1.23** | 311 | 211.06 | 1.47** |
| RECTUM | 304 | 256.46 | 1.19** | 45 | 52.54 | 0.86 | 129 | 100.58 | 1.28** | 130 | 103.34 | 1.26** |
| LUNG AND BRONCHUS | 331 | 278.00 | 1.19** | 28 | 61.52 | 0.46** | 140 | 112.07 | 1.25** | 163 | 104.41 | 1.56** |
| OTHER RESP | 9 | 5.04 | 1.78 | 2 | 1.15 | 1.75 | 0 | 2.04 | 0.0 | 7 | 1.86 | 3.77** |
| BREAST | 944 | 492.64 | 1.92** | 157 | 84.86 | 1.85** | 404 | 186.11 | 2.17** | 383 | 221.67 | 1.73** |
| CORPUS UTERI | 157 | 104.99 | 1.50** | 25 | 17.21 | 1.45 | 61 | 38.79 | 1.57** | 71 | 48.98 | 1.45** |
| OVARY | 172 | 97.19 | 1.77** | 41 | 16.78 | 2.44** | 65 | 36.98 | 1.76** | 66 | 43.43 | 1.52** |
| OTHER FEMALE GENITAL | 39 | 20.82 | 1.87** | 4 | 3.45 | 1.16 | 13 | 7.59 | 1.71 | 22 | 9.78 | 2.25** |
| PROSTATE | 459 | 342.80 | 1.34** | 144 | 76.05 | 1.89** | 154 | 139.13 | 1.11 | 161 | 127.61 | 1.26** |
| TESTIS | 12 | 3.59 | 3.34** | 6 | 0.91 | 6.61** | 4 | 1.52 | 2.62 | 2 | 1.16 | 1.72 |
| KIDNEY AND URETER | 119 | 69.10 | 1.72** | 44 | 14.11 | 3.12** | 40 | 27.09 | 1.48* | 35 | 27.90 | 1.25 |
| BLADDER | 239 | 189.25 | 1.26** | 39 | 39.75 | 0.98 | 126 | 74.63 | 1.69** | 74 | 74.87 | 0.99 |
| MELANOMA OF SKIN | 45 | 26.01 | 1.73** | 14 | 5.02 | 2.79** | 19 | 10.14 | 1.87* | 12 | 10.85 | 1.11 |
| EYE | 15 | 7.15 | 2.10* | 4 | 1.46 | 2.74 | 6 | 2.81 | 2.13 | 5 | 2.87 | 1.74 |
| THYROID | 30 | 20.32 | 1.48 | 13 | 3.76 | 3.46** | 6 | 7.84 | 0.77 | 11 | 8.73 | 1.26 |
| SOFT TISSUE | 48 | 24.08 | 1.99** | 11 | 4.68 | 2.35* | 15 | 9.28 | 1.62 | 22 | 10.11 | 2.18** |
| LEUKEMIAS | 118 | 100.85 | 1.17 | 19 | 20.00 | 0.95 | 45 | 38.98 | 1.15 | 54 | 41.87 | 1.29 |

Table 137. Subsequent primary sites with deficiencies (excluding non-melanotic skin cancer)

FIRST PRIMARY - ALL SITES (excluding non-melanotic skin cancer)

| | TOTAL | | | YEARS < 1 | | | YEARS 1-5 | | | YEARS > 5 | | |
|---|---|---|---|---|---|---|---|---|---|---|---|---|
| | NUMBER OF PERSONS=121460 PERSON-YRS OF OBSERVATION= 419382.9 | | | NUMBER OF PERSONS=121460 PERSON-YRS OF OBSERVATION= 88408.9 | | | NUMBER OF PERSONS= 69292 PERSON-YRS OF OBSERVATION= 170850.1 | | | NUMBER OF PERSONS= 27551 PERSON-YRS OF OBSERVATION= 160123.9 | | |
| SUBSEQUENT PRIMARY SITES | OBS | EXP | OBS/EXP | OBS | EXP | OBS/EXP | OBS | EXP | OBS/EXP | OBS | EXP | OBS/EXP |
| STOMACH | 227 | 305.98 | 0.74** | 43 | 65.92 | 0.65** | 99 | 121.76 | 0.81* | 85 | 118.31 | 0.72** |
| PANCREAS | 116 | 130.56 | 0.89 | 35 | 26.02 | 1.35 | 48 | 50.39 | 0.95 | 33 | 54.15 | 0.61** |
| NERVOUS SYSTEM | 21 | 33.90 | 0.62* | 4 | 7.24 | 0.55 | 9 | 13.73 | 0.66 | 8 | 12.94 | 0.62 |
| OTHER SITES | 168 | 211.34 | 0.79** | 28 | 40.60 | 0.69* | 65 | 80.46 | 0.81 | 75 | 90.29 | 0.83 |

Table 138. Histologic confirmation of multiple primary malignancies

FIRST PRIMARY SITE - ALL SITES (excluding non-melanotic skin cancer)

| Subsequent primary site | Both tumors microscopically confirmed | | Only 1st tumor microscopically confirmed | | Only 2nd tumor microscopically confirmed | | Neither tumor microscopically confirmed | |
|---|---|---|---|---|---|---|---|---|
| | No. | % | No. | % | No. | % | No. | % |
| LIP | 36 | 83.7 | 5 | 11.6 | 2 | 4.7 | 0 | 0.0 |
| TONGUE | 57 | 80.3 | 6 | 8.5 | 7 | 9.9 | 1 | 1.4 |
| MOUTH | 73 | 92.4 | 1 | 1.3 | 3 | 3.8 | 2 | 2.5 |
| PHARYNX | 53 | 81.5 | 6 | 9.2 | 5 | 7.7 | 1 | 1.5 |
| ESOPHAGUS | 58 | 77.3 | 10 | 13.3 | 5 | 6.7 | 2 | 2.7 |
| SMALL INTESTINE | 22 | 95.7 | 0 | 0.0 | 1 | 4.3 | 0 | 0.0 |
| COLON | 550 | 84.0 | 71 | 10.8 | 25 | 3.8 | 9 | 1.4 |
| RECTUM | 253 | 83.2 | 31 | 10.2 | 14 | 4.6 | 6 | 2.0 |
| LUNG AND BRONCHUS | 248 | 74.9 | 58 | 17.5 | 14 | 4.2 | 11 | 3.3 |
| OTHER RESP | 6 | 66.7 | 3 | 33.3 | 0 | 0.0 | 0 | 0.0 |
| BREAST | 829 | 87.8 | 52 | 5.5 | 53 | 5.6 | 10 | 1.1 |
| CORPUS UTERI | 144 | 91.7 | 4 | 2.5 | 6 | 3.8 | 3 | 1.9 |
| OVARY | 156 | 90.7 | 6 | 3.5 | 10 | 5.8 | 0 | 0.0 |
| OTHER FEMALE GENITAL | 37 | 94.9 | 1 | 2.6 | 0 | 0.0 | 1 | 2.6 |
| PROSTATE | 348 | 75.8 | 79 | 17.2 | 19 | 4.1 | 13 | 2.8 |
| TESTIS | 12 | 100.0 | 0 | 0.0 | 0 | 0.0 | 0 | 0.0 |
| KIDNEY AND URETER | 95 | 79.8 | 14 | 11.8 | 9 | 7.6 | 1 | 0.8 |
| BLADDER | 188 | 78.7 | 29 | 12.1 | 16 | 6.7 | 6 | 2.5 |
| MELANOMA OF SKIN | 43 | 95.6 | 0 | 0.0 | 2 | 4.4 | 0 | 0.0 |
| EYE | 14 | 93.3 | 0 | 0.0 | 0 | 0.0 | 1 | 6.7 |
| THYROID | 26 | 86.7 | 1 | 3.3 | 2 | 6.7 | 1 | 3.3 |
| SOFT TISSUE | 44 | 91.7 | 1 | 2.1 | 2 | 4.2 | 1 | 2.1 |
| LEUKEMIAS | 94 | 79.7 | 14 | 11.9 | 7 | 5.9 | 3 | 2.5 |

# References


1. ACHESON, R.M., CHAPPLE, M., EISENBERG, H.: Infertility as a risk factor for carcinoma of the colon in women. Submitted for publication
2. ANDERSON, D.E.: Familial susceptibility. In: Persons at High Risk of Cancer: An Approach to Cancer Etiology and Control. J.F. Fraumeni, Jr., (ed.) New York: Academic Press, 1975, pp. 39-55
3. ARSENEAU, J.C., SPONZO, R.W., LEVIN, D.L., et al.: Nonlymphomatous malignant tumors complicating Hodgkin's disease: Possible association with intensive therapy. N. Engl. J. Med. 287, 1119-1122 (1972)
4. AUSTIN, R.S.: Multiple primary malignant tumors. Scientific Proceedings of the Thirty-Eighth Annual Meeting of the American Association of Pathologists and Bacteriologists. Amer. J. Path. 14, 664-667 (1938)
5. BAILAR, J.C., III: The incidence of independent tumors among uterine cancer patients. Cancer 16, 842-853 (1963)
6. BAILAR, J.C., III, EDERER, F.: Significance factors for the ratio of a Poisson variable to its expectation. Biometrics 20, 639-643 (1964)
7. BAUGHMAN, F.A., Jr., LIST, C.F., WILLIAMS, J.R., et al.: The glioma-polyposis syndrome. N. Engl. J. Med. 281, 1345-1346 (1969)
8. BENISCH, B.M., TOKER, C.: The coexistence of an ovarian Brenner tumor and endometrial stromal sarcoma. Mt. Sinai J. Med. N.Y. 40, 689-692 (1973)
9. BERG, J.W.: The incidence of multiple primary cancers. I. Development of further cancers in patients with lymphomas, leukemias, and myeloma. J. Natl. Cancer Inst. 38, 741-753 (1967)
10. BERG, J.W., HUTTER, R.V.P., FOOTE, F.W., Jr.: The unique association between salivary gland cancer and breast cancer. J.A.M.A. 204, 771-774 (1968)
11. BERG, J.W., SCHOTTENFELD, D., RITTER, F.: Incidence of multiple primary cancers. III. Cancers of the respiratory and upper digestive system as multiple primary cancers. J. Natl. Cancer Inst. 44, 263-274 (1970)
12. BERGE, T., CEDERQVIST, L., SCHÖNEBECK, J.: Multiple primary malignant tumours: An autopsy study of a circumscribed population. Acta path. microbiol. Scand., 76, 171-183 (1969)
13. BLOOMFIELD, R.D., SAMIMY, J.B.: Multiple primary malignancies of the female genital tract. J. Natl. Med. Assoc. 64, 230-231 (1972)
14. BUGHER, J.C.: The probability of the chance occurrence of multiple malignant neoplasms. Amer. J. Cancer 21, 809-824 (1934)
15. BURKE, M.: Multiple primary cancers. Amer. J. Cancer 27, 316-325 (1936)
16. CAHAN, W.G.: Multiple primary cancers, one of which is lung. Surg. Clin. N. Amer. 49, 323-325 (1969)

17. CAHAN, W.G., MONTEMAYOR, P.B.: Cancer of the larynx and lung in the same patient: A report of 60 cases. J. Thoracic Cardiovasc. Surg. 44, 309-320 (1962)
18. CASTIGLIANO, S.G.: Influence of continued smoking on the incidence of second primary cancers involving mouth, pharynx, and larynx. J. Am. Dent. Assoc. 77, 580-585 (1968)
19. CONNELLY, R.R., CAMPBELL, P.C., EISENBERG, H.: Central registry of cancer cases in Connecticut. Public Health Rep. 83, 386-390 (1968)
20. COOPER, Z.: Discussion. In: Multiple skin cancer; a statistical and pathological study. Phillips, C. Southern Med. J. 35, 583-588 (1942)
21. CORI, C.F.: The influence of ovariectomy on the spontaneous occurrence of mammary carcinomas in mice. J. Exp. Med. 45, 983-991 (1927)
22. CORSCADEN, J.A.: Gynecologic Cancer, 3rd. ed., Baltimore: Williams & Wilkins, Co., 1962, p. 333
23. DENCKER, H., LIEDBERG, G., TIBBLIN, S.: Multiple malignant tumors of the colon and rectum. Acta Chir. Scand. 135, 260-262 (1969)
24. DEVITT, J.E., ROTH-MOYO, L.A., BROWN, F.N.: The significance of multiple adenocarcinomas of the colon and rectum. Ann. Surg. 169, 364-367 (1969)
25. DOCKERTY, M.B., LOVELADY, S.B., FOUST, G.T., Jr.: Carcinoma of the corpus uteri in young women. Am. J. Obstet. Gynecol. 61, 966-981 (1955)
26. DOLL, R., HILL, A.B.: Mortality in relation to smoking: Ten years' observations of British doctors. Br. Med. J. 1, 1399-1410 (1964)
27. DUNHAM, L.J., BAILAR, J.C., III: World maps of cancer mortality rates and frequency ratios. J. Natl. Cancer Inst. 41, 155-201 (1968)
28. DUNN, J.E., BRAGG, K.U., SAUTTER, C., et al.: Breast cancer risk following a major salivary gland carcinoma. Cancer 29, 1343-1346 (1972)
29. EDITORIAL. Hazard of mineral-oil mist? Lancet II, 967-968 (1970)
30. EINHORN, J., JAKOBSSON, L.: Multiple primary malignant tumors. Cancer 17, 1437-1444 (1964)
31. EISENBERG, H.: Cancer in Connecticut; Incidence and Rates 1935-1952. Hartford, Conn.: Conn. State Dept. of Health, 1966.
32. END RESULTS SECTION, NATIONAL CANCER INSTITUTE: 1967 Code Manual of the End Results Group. Washington, D.C.: U.S. Government Printing Office, 1967, 217 pp
33. EPSTEIN, E.: Association of mucocutaneous and visceral cancers. Arch. Derm. Syph. 69, 58-65 (1954)
34. FISHER, J.C., KETCHAM, A.S.: Multiple primary malignancies: A critical review. W. Virginia Med. J. 62, 137-139 (1966)
35. FRAUMENI, J.F., Jr.: Genetic factors. In: Cancer Medicine. Holland, J.F., Frei, E., III, (eds.) Philadelphia: Lea & Febiger, 1973, pp. 7-15
36. FRAUMENI, J.F., Jr., LLOYD, J.W., SMITH, E.M., et al.: Cancer mortality among nuns: Role of marital status in etiology of neoplastic disease in women. J. Natl. Cancer Inst. 42, 455-468 (1969)
37. FRIED, D.M.: Primary double cancer. Arch. Path. 5, 565-578 (1928)
38. FRIED, D.M.: Primary multiple cancers. A.M.A. Arch. Surg. 77, 730-741 (1958)
39. GARDNER, E.J., RICHARDS, R.C.: Multiple cutaneous and subcutaneous lesions occurring simultaneously with hereditary polyposis and osteomatosis. Am. J. Hum. Genet. 5, 139-147 (1953)
40. GILLIAM, A.G.: Fertility and cancer of the breast and uterine cervix: Comparisons between rates of pregnancy in women with cancer at these and other sites. J. Natl. Cancer Inst. 12, 287-304 (1951)
41. GREENBERG, R.A.: The Connecticut tumor registry. Conn. Health Bull. 73, 35-42 (1959a)

42. GREENBERG, R.A.: The Occurrence of Primary Multiple Cancers. Thesis. New Haven: Yale University, 1959b, 27 pp
43. GUERRIER, K.R., PERSKY, L.: Combined leukemia, carcinoma, and hyperplasia of the prostate. Arch. Surg. 98, 365-366 (1969)
44. HAJDU, S.I., HAJDU, E.O.: Multiple primary malignant tumors. J. Amer. Geriat. Soc. 16, 16-26 (1968)
45. HAMMOND, E.C.: Smoking in relation to the death rates of one million men and women. Natl. Cancer Inst. Monogr. 19, 127-204 (1966)
46. HAMMOND, E.C.: Tobacco. In: Persons At High Risk of Cancer: An Approach to Cancer Etiology and Control. Fraumeni, J.F., Jr. (ed.) New York: Academic Press, 1975, pp. 131-138
47. HAMMOND, E.C., HORN, D.: Smoking and death rates - report of forty-four months of follow-up of 187,183 men. Part II. Death rates by cause. J.A.M.A. 166, 1294-1308 (1958)
48. HANLON, F.R.: Multiple primary carcinomas. Amer. J. Cancer 15, 2001-2011 (1931)
49. HARNETT, W.L.: A statistical report on 2529 cases of cancer of the breast. Br. J. Cancer 2, 212-239 (1948)
50. HAUSER, I.J., WELLER, C.V.: A further report on the cancer family of Warthin. Am. J. Cancer 27, 434-449 (1936)
51. HEIBERG, B., HEIBERG, P.: Some investigations into the occurrence of carcinoma of the breast with special reference to the ovarian function. Acta Chir. Scand. 83, 479-496 (1940)
52. HELLENDALL, H.: Multiple carcinoma: The clinical picture, diagnosis and prognosis. Amer. J. Surg. 60, 22-35 (1943)
53. HIGGINSON, J., MUIR, C.S.: Epidemiology. In: Cancer Medicine, Holland, J.F., Frei, E., III (eds.) Philadelphia: Lea & Febiger, 1973, pp. 258-275
54. HOLLAND, J.F., FREI, E., III, eds.: Cancer Medicine. Philadelphia: Lea & Febiger, 1973, pp. 1173-1199; 1425-1879
55. HOLMES, J.G., KIPLING, M.D., WATERHOUSE, J.A.H.: Subsequent malignancies in men with scrotal epithelioma. Lancet II, 214-215 (1970)
56. HURT, H.H., BRODERS, A.C.: Multiple primary malignant neoplasms. J. Lab. Clin. Med. 18, 765-777 (1933)
57. JABLON, S.: Radiation. In: Persons At High Risk of Cancer: An Approach to Cancer Etiology and Control. Fraumeni, J.F., Jr., (ed.) New York: Academic Press, 1975, pp. 151-165
58. JENSEN, R.D., MILLER, R.W.: Retinoblastoma: epidemiologic characteristics. N. Engl. J. Med. 285, 307-311 (1971)
59. JIMERSON, G.K., MERRILL, J.A.: Multicentric squamous malignancy involving both cervix and vulva. Cancer 26, 150-153 (1970)
60. JOHNSON, G.J., SUMMERSKILL, W.H.J., ANDERSON, V.E., et al.: Clinical and genetic investigation of a large kindred with multiple endocrine adenomatosis. N. Engl. J. Med. 277, 1379-1385 (1967)
61. KARCHMER, R.K., AMARE, M., LARSON, W.E., et al.: Alkylating agents as leukemogens in multiple myeloma. Cancer 33, 1103-1107 (1974)
62. KELLER, A.Z., TERRIS, M.: The association of alcohol and tobacco with cancer of the mouth and pharynx. Am. J. Public Health 55, 1578-1585 (1965)
63. KERSEY, J.H., SPECTOR, B.D., GOOD, R.A.: Primary immunodeficiency diseases and cancer: The immunodeficiency-cancer registry. Int. J. Cancer 12, 333-347 (1973)
64. KILGORE, A.R.J.: The incidence of cancer in the second breast after radical removal of one breast for cancer. J.A.M.A. 77, 454-457 (1921)
65. KIRSHBAUM, J.D., SHIVELY, F.L., Jr.: Multiple primary malignant tumors. J. Lab. Clin. Med. 24, 283-292 (1938)
66. KITCHIN, P.D., ELLSWORTH, R.M.: Pleiotropic effects of the gene for retinoblastoma. J. Med. Genet. 11, 244-246 (1974)

67. LEVIN, D.L., DEVESA, S.S., GODWIN, J.D., II, et al.: Cancer Rates and Risks, 2nd ed. Washington, D.C.: U.S. Government Printing Office, 1974, 108 pp
68. LILIENFELD, A.M.: The epidemiology of breast cancer. Cancer Res. 23, 1503-1513 (1963)
69. LILIENFELD, A.M., LEVIN, M.L., MOORE, G.E.: The association of smoking with cancer of the urinary bladder in humans. Arch. Int. Med. 98, 129-135 (1956)
70. LOMBARD, H.L., WARREN, S.: Association of other malignant tumors with cancer of the skin. Amer. J. Public Health 35, 533-536 (1943)
71. LOMBARD, H.L., LEVIN, M.L., WARREN, S.: Multiple malignant growths. Cancer Res. 6, 436-440 (1946)
72. LUND, C.C.: Second primary cancer in cases of cancer of the buccal mucosa; a mathematical study of susceptibility to cancer. New Engl. J. Med. 209, 1144-1152 (1933)
73. LYNCH, H.T., LARSEN, A.L., MAGNUSON, C.W., et al.: Prostate carcinoma and multiple primary malignancies. Cancer 19, 1891-1897 (1966)
74. LYNCH, H.T., KRUSH, A.J., LARSEN, A.L.: Heredity and multiple primary malignant neoplasms: Six cancer families. Am. J. Med. Sci. 254, 322-329 (1967)
75. MACDONALD, E.J.: Occurrence of multiple primary cancers in a population of 200,000. Acta Un. Int. Cancr. 16, 1702-1711 (1960)
76. MACMAHON, B., AUSTIN, J.H.: Association of carcinomas of the breast and corpus uteri. Cancer 23, 275-280 (1969)
77. MACMAHON, C.E., ROWE, J.W.: Rectal reaction following radiation therapy of cervical carcinoma: Particular reference to subsequent occurrence of rectal carcinoma. Ann. Surg. 173, 264-269 (1971)
78. MAJOR, R.H.: Multiple primary malignant tumors with report of a case of carcinoma and sarcoma in the same individual. Bull. Hopkins Hosp. 29, 223-231 (1918)
79. MALMIO, K.: Multiple primary cancer; a clinical statistical investigation based on 650 cases. Ann. Chir. Gynaec. Fenn. (Suppl. 92) 48, 1-124 (1959)
80. MARCUSE, P.M.: Diagnostic Pathology in Gynecology and Obstetrics. New York & London: Harper & Row (Hoeber Medical Division), 1966, pp. 14, 143
81. MEDICAL COMMITTEE OF THE SOCIETY FOR INVESTIGATING THE NATURE AND CURE OF CANCER: "Report." Edin. Med. & Surg. J. 2, 383-389 (1806)
82. MICHELSEN, J., NEW, P.F.I.: Brain tumour and pregnancy J. Neurol. Neurosurg. Psychiatry 32, 305-307 (1969)
83. MIDER, G.B.: Multiple invasive carcinomas of the large intestine. Surgery 20, 744-748 (1946)
84. MOERTEL, C.G.: Multiple Primary Malignant Neoplasms: Their Incidence and Significance. Berlin-Heidelberg-New York: Springer-Verlag, 1966, 108 pp
85. MOERTEL, C.G., ELVEBACK, L.R.: The association between salivary gland cancer and breast cancer. J.A.M.A. 210, 306-308 (1969)
86. MOERTEL, C.G., DOCKERTY, M.B., BAGGENSTOSS, A.H.: Multiple primary malignant neoplasms. I. Introduction and presentation of data. II. Tumors of different tissues or organs. Cancer 14, 221-237 (1961)
87. MOORE, C.: Cigarette smoking and cancer of the mouth, pharynx, and larynx. J.A.M.A. 218, 553-558 (1971)
88. MORIARTY, M.: Skin carcinoma and chronic lymphatic leukemia - An association. J. Irish Med. Assoc. 67, 177-180 (1974)
89. MORRIS, J. McL., SCULLY, R.E.: Endocrine Pathology of the Ovary. St. Louis: C.V. Mosby Co., 1958, p. 53
90. MORTON, R.F., VILLASANTA, U.: New cancers arising in 1,563 patients with carcinoma of the cervix treated by irradiation. Am. J. Obstet. Gynecol. 115, 462-466 (1973)

91. MUSTAKALLIO, S.: Cutaneous cancer in Finland; clinical and radiotherapeutic study of 1,068 cases. Ann. Chir. Gynaec. Fenn. (Suppl. 3) 35, 1-95 (1946)
92. NEWELL, G.R., KREMENTZ, E.T., ROBERTS, J.D., et al.: Multiple primary neoplasms in blacks compared to whites. I. Further cancers in patients with Hodgkin's disease, leukemia, and myeloma. J. Natl. Cancer Inst. 52, 635-638 (1974a)
93. NEWELL, G.R., KREMENTZ, E.T., ROBERTS, J.D.: Multiple primary neoplasms in blacks compared to whites. II. Further cancers in patients with cancer of the buccal cavity and pharynx. J. Natl. Cancer Inst. 52, 639-642 (1974b)
94. NEWELL, G.R., RAWLINGS, W., KREMENTZ, E.T., et al.: Multiple primary neoplasms in blacks compared to whites. III. Initial cancers of the female breast and uterus. J. Natl. Cancer Inst. 53, 369-373 (1974c)
95. NEWELL, G.R., KREMENTZ, E.T., ROBERTS, J.D.: Multiple primary neoplasms in blacks compared to whites. IV. Further cancers in patients with cancer of the digestive organs. J. Natl. Cancer Inst. 54, 331-334 (1975)
96. NOVAK, E.R., WOODRUFF, J.D.: Postirradiation malignancies of the pelvic organs. Am. J. Obstet. Gynecol. 77, 667-675 (1959)
97. OLCH, I.Y.: Menopausal age in women with cancer of the breast. Am. J. Cancer 30, 565-566 (1937)
98. ORR, J.W.: Multiple malignant neoplasms. J. Path. Bact. 33, 283-290 (1930)
99. PEARSON, E.S., HARTLEY, H.O.: Biometrika Tables for Statisticians, 2nd ed. Cambridge: Cambridge University Press, 1958, Vol. I, p. 203
100. PEARSON, J.: Practical Observations on Cancerous Complaints: With An Account of Some Diseases Which Have Been Confounded With the Cancer; Also, Critical Remarks on Some of the Operations Performed in Cancerous Cases. London, 1793
101. PELLER, S.: Metachronous multiple malignancies in 5,876 cancer patients. Amer. J. Hyg. 34, 1-11 (1941)
102. PENN, I., STARZL, T.E.: A summary of the status of de novo cancer in transplant recipients. Transplant. Proc. 4, 719 (1972)
103. PHILLIPS, C.: Multiple skin cancer; a statistical and pathological study. Southern Med. J. 35, 583-588 (1942)
104. PICKREN, J.W.: Cancer often strikes twice. New York J. Med. 63, 95-99 (1963)
105. POLK, H.C., Jr., SPRATT, J.S., Jr., BUTCHER, H.R.: Frequency of multiple primary malignant neoplasms associated with colorectal carcinoma. Am. J. Surg. 109, 71-75 (1965)
106. QIZILBASH, A.H.: Radiation-induced carcinoma of the rectum: A late complication of pelvic irradiation. Arch. Pathol. 98, 118-121 (1974)
107. RAJHAVJN, B., KURJAK, A.: Multiple primary neoplasms in gynecology. Acta Med. Iugosl. 27, 369-374 (1973)
108. ROBBINS, G.F., BERG, J.W.: Bilateral primary breast cancer: A prospective clinicopathological study. Cancer 17, 1501-1537 (1964)
109. ROTHMAN, K.J.: Alcohol. In: Persons At High Risk of Cancer: An Approach to Cancer Etiology and Control. Fraumeni, J.F., Jr., (ed.) New York: Academic Press, 1975, pp. 139-150
110. RUBIN, P., ed.: Clinical Oncology for Medical Students and Physicians: A Multidisciplinary Approach, 4th ed. Rochester, N.Y.: American Cancer Society, 1974, pp. 129-486
111. RUBINSTEIN, L.J.: Tumors of the Central Nervous System. Atlas of Tumor Pathology, 2nd. series, Fasc. 6. Washington, D.C.: Armed Forces Institute of Pathology, 1972, pp. 302-303
112. SAVAGE, D.: A family history of uterine and gastrointestinal cancer. Br. Med. J. 2, 341-343 (1956)

113. SCHIMKE, R.N., HARTMANN, W.H., PROUT, T.E., et al.: Syndrome of bilateral pheochromocytoma, medullary thyroid carcinoma, and multiple neuromas. N. Engl. J. Med. 279, 1-7 (1966)
114. SCHOENBERG, B.S.: The unique association between meningiomas and breast cancer (abstract). Neurology 24, 356 (1974)
115. SCHOENBERG, B.S.: A program for the conquest of cancer: 1802. J. Hist. Med. & Allied Sci. 30, 1-22 (1975)
116. SCHOENBERG, B.S., CHRISTINE, B.W.: The association of neoplasms of the colon and rectum with primary malignancies of other sites. Am. J. Proctol. 25, 41-60 (1974)
117. SCHOENBERG, B.S., CHRISTINE, B.W.: Gynecologic malignancies associated with other primary malignant neoplasms. Submitted for publication
118. SCHOENBERG, B.S., GREENBERG, R.A., EISENBERG, H.: Occurrence of certain multiple primary cancers in females. J. Natl. Cancer Inst. 43, 15-32 (1969)
119. SCHOENBERG, B.S., BAILAR, J.C., III., FRAUMENI, J.F., Jr.: Certain mortality patterns of esophageal cancer in the United States, 1930-67. J. Natl. Cancer Inst. 46, 63-73 (1971)
120. SCHOENBERG, B.S., CHRISTINE, B.W., WHISNANT, J.P.: Nervous system neoplasms and primary malignancies of other sites. The unique association between meningiomas and breast cancer. Neurology 25, 705-712 (1975)
121. SCHOENBERG, B.S., CHRISTINE, B.W., WHISNANT, J.P.: The descriptive epidemiology of primary intracranial neoplasms: The Connecticut experience. Am. J. Epid. 104, 499-510, 1976
122. SCHOTTENFELD, D., BERG, J.W.: Incidence of multiple primary cancers. IV. Cancers of the female breast and genital organs. J. Natl. Cancer Inst. 46, 161-170 (1971)
123. SCHOTTENFELD, D., BERG, J.W., VITSKY, B.: Incidence of multiple primary cancers. II. Index cancers arising in the stomach and lower digestive system. J. Natl. Cancer Inst. 43, 77-86 (1969)
124. SCHOTTENFELD, D., GANTT, R.C., WYNDER, E.L.: The role of alcohol and tobacco in multiple primary cancers of the upper digestive system, larynx, and lung: A prospective study. Prev. Med. 3, 277-293 (1974)
125. SCHREINER, B.F., WEHR, W.H.: Multiple primary cancer as observed at the State Institute for the Study of Malignant Disease. Amer. J. Cancer 20, 418-424 (1934)
126. SILVERMAN, B.B., O'NEILL, R.T., MIKUTA, J.J.: Multiple malignant tumors associated with primary carcinoma of the ovary. Surg. Gynec. Obstet. 134, 244-248 (1972)
127. SLAUGHTER, D.P.: Multiplicity of origin of malignant tumors; collective review. Int. Abstr. Surg. 79, 89-98 (1944)
128. SLAUGHTER, D.P., SOUTHWICK, H.W.: Mucosal carcinoma as a result of irradiation. Arch. Surg. 74, 420-429 (1957)
129. SMITH, J.C.: Carcinoma of the rectum following irradiation of carcinoma of the cervix. Proc. Roy. Soc. Med. 55, 701-702 (1962)
130. SOMMERS, S.C., HERTIG, A.T., BENGLOFF, H.: Genesis of endometrial carcinoma. II. Cases 19 to 35 years old. Cancer 2, 957-963 (1949)
131. SOUADJIAN, J.V., SILVERSTEIN, M.N., TITUS, J.: Thymoma and cancer. Cancer 22, 1221-1225 (1968)
132. SPEERT, H.: Carcinoma of the endometrium in young women. Surg. Gynec. Obstet. 88, 332-336 (1949)
133. SPRATT, J.S., Jr., HOAG, M.G.: Incidence of multiple primary cancers per man-year of follow-up; 20-year review from the Ellis Fischel State Cancer Hospital. Ann. Surg. 164, 775-784 (1966)
134. STALKER, L.K., PHILLIPS, R.B., PEMBERTON, J. deJ.: Multiple primary malignant lesions. Surg. Gynec. Obstet. 68, 595-602 (1939)
135. STEINITZ, R.: Five-Years' Morbidity from Neoplasms in Israel's Population Groups (1960-1964), Ministry of Health, Division of Chronic Diseases and Rehabilitation, Jerusalem, Israel, 1967

136. STEWART, F.W., TREVES, N.: Lymphangiosarcoma in postmastectomy lymphedema: report of 6 cases in elephantiasis chirurgica. Cancer 1, 64-81 (1948)
137. THOMA, G.W.: The incidence and significance of multiple primary malignant tumors; a study of 2346 necropsies from a cancer research hospital. Amer. J. Med. Sci. 247, 427-430 (1964)
138. TRAVIESO, C.R., KNOEPP, L.F., Jr., HANLEY, P.H.: Multiple adenocarcinomas of the colon and rectum. Dis. Colon Rectum 15, 1-6 (1972)
139. TULLIS, J.L.: Multiple primary malignant lesions. J. Lab. Clin. Med. 27, 588-594 (1942)
140. TURCOT, J., DESPRES, J.P., ST. PIERRE, F.: Malignant tumors of the central nervous system associated with familial polyposis of the colon: Report of two cases. Dis. Colon Rectum 2, 465-468 (1959)
141. VONGTAMA, V., KUROHARA, S.S., BADIB, A.O., et al.: Second primary cancers of endometrial carcinoma. Cancer 26, 842-846 (1970)
142. WALL, R.S., CLAUSEN, K.P.: Carcinoma of the urinary bladder in patients receiving cyclophosphamide. N. Engl. J. Med. 293, 271-273 (1975)
143. WARREN, S., EHRENREICH, T.: Multiple primary malignant tumors and susceptibility to cancer. Cancer Res. 4, 554-570 (1944)
144. WARREN, S., GATES, O.: Multiple primary malignant tumors; a survey of the literature and statistical study. Amer. J. Cancer 16, 1358-1414 (1932)
145. WARREN, S., GATES, O.: Cancer of the skin in relation to multiple malignant growths. J.A.M.A. 115, 1705-1707 (1940)
146. WATSON, T.A.: Incidence of multiple cancer. Cancer 6, 365-371 (1953)
147. WELLS, H.G.: Multiple primary malignant tumors; report of a primary sarco-carcinoma in the thyroid of a dog, with mixed sarcomatous and carcinomatous metastasis. J. Path. Bact. 7, 357-367 (1901)
148. WILLIS, R.S.: The Spread of Tumours in the Human Body, 3rd. ed. London: Butterworth & Co., Ltd., 1973, 417 pp
149. WILLSON, J.R., BEECHAM, C.T., CARRINGTON, E.R.: Obstetrics and Gynecology, 2nd ed. St. Louis: C.V. Mosby Co., 1963, pp. 631-633
150. WOODRUFF, J.D., JULIAN, C.G.: Multiple malignancy in the upper genital canal. Am. J. Obstet. Gynecol. 103, 810-822 (1969)
151. WOOLLEY, P.G.: Notes on multiple primary tumors. Boston Med. Surg. J. 148, 1-6 (1903)
152. WORLD HEALTH ORGANIZATION: International Classification of Diseases. Manual of the International Statistical Classification of Diseases, Injuries, and Causes of Death. Vol. 1. Geneva, Switzerland, 1957, 393 pp
153. WYNDER, E.L., BROSS, I.J.: A study of etiological factors in cancer of the esophagus. Cancer 14, 389-413 (1961)
154. WYNDER, E.L., BROSS, I.J., HIRAYAMA, T.: A study of the epidemiology of cancer of the breast. Cancer 13, 559-601 (1960)
155. WYNDER, E.L., HYAMS, L., SHIGEMATSU, T.: Correlations of international cancer rates; an epidemiological exercise. Cancer 20, 113-126 (1967)
156. WYNDER, E.L., DODO, H., BLOCH, D., et al.: Epidemiologic investigation of multiple primary cancer of the upper alimentary and respiratory tracts. I. A retrospective study. Cancer 24, 730-739 (1969)

Additional References


HARRIS, C.C.: The carcinogenicity of anticancer drugs; a hazard in man. Cancer 37, 1014-1023 (1976)

HODGIN, J.D., WEBSTER, P.D.: Malignancies in blood-forming organs following diagnostic and therapeutic procedures; a review. South. Med. J. 69, 1363-1366 (1976)

HUTCHISON, G.B.: Late neoplastic changes following medical irradiation. Cancer 37, 1102-1107 (1976)

JOCHIMSEN, P.R., BROWN, R.C.: Metastatic melanoma in the breast masquerading as fibroadenoma. J.A.M.A. 236, 2779-2780 (1976)

KIPLING, M.D., WALDRON, H.A.: Polycyclic aromatic hydrocarbons in mineral oil, tar, and pitch, excluding petroleum pitch. Prev. Med. 5, 262-278 (1976)

PENN, I.: Second malignant neoplasms associated with immuno-suppressive medications. Cancer 37, 1024-1032 (1976)

ROSNER, F.: Acute leukemia as a delayed consequence of cancer chemotherapy. Cancer 37, 1033-1036 (1976)

VAISMAN, I., BELLET, R.E., MASTRANGELO, M.J., et al.: Multiple primary malignancies in patients with cutaneous melanoma (abstract). In: International Workshop on Multiple Primary Cancers. CAHAN, W.G., SCHOTTENFELD, D., MOERTEL, C.G., (eds.) New York: Memorial Sloan-Kettering Cancer Center, 1976

WILLIAMS, R.R.: Breast and thyroid cancer and malignant melanoma promoted by alcohol-induced pituitary secretion of prolactin, T.S.H., and M.S.H. Lancet 1, 996-999 (1976)

# Appendix

Only malignant neoplasms were included in analyses presented in this monograph. The Connecticut Tumor Registry defines malignancy as follows (END RESULTS SECTION, NATIONAL CANCER INSTITUTE, 1967):

> This category includes diagnoses commonly accepted as denoting malignancy, or specified by the word "malignant" in the diagnostic phrase, or otherwise considered malignant at the reporting (hospital) registries.
>
> Among the diagnoses accepted as malignant without use of the word "malignant" are the following: Diagnoses containing terms or suffixes like carcinoma, sarcoma, blastoma, leukemia, cancer of ...... or containing the associated adjectives carcinomatous, sarcomatous, leukemic, cancerous, etc. Note, however, that there are a few exceptions such as "cystosarcoma phyllodes" which require additional specification by the word "malignant" to be considered as cancer.

Anatomic sites are defined as follows with reference to corresponding code numbers in the Seventh Revision of the <u>International Classification of Diseases</u> (WORLD HEALTH ORGANIZATION, 1957):

| ICD CODE | SITE DESIGNATION |
|---|---|
| (International Classification of Diseases) | I. Buccal Cavity and Pharynx |
| | A. Lip (labial mucosa), excluding "skin of lip" |
| 140.0 | upper lip, not specified as midline |
| 140.1 | lower lip, not specified as midline |
| 140.3 | commissure |
| 140.5 | upper lip, midline tumor |
| 140.6 | lower lip, midline tumor |
| 140.9 | lip, unspecified (including "both lips," not otherwise specified, with site of primary not determined) |
| | B. Tongue |
| | Base of tongue (tongue posterior to circumvallate papillae. Includes "posterior third", not otherwise specified.) |
| 141.0 | midline tumor |
| 141.1 | other than midline, and "base not otherwise specified" |

| ICD CODE | SITE DESIGNATION |
|---|---|
| | Anterior two-thirds of tongue (tongue anterior to circumvallate papillae) |
| | dorsal surface of tongue (top) |
| 141.2 | midline tumor |
| 141.3 | other than midline, and "dorsal," not otherwise specified |
| | ventral surface of tongue (underside) |
| 141.4 | midline tumor |
| 141.5 | other than midline, and "underside," not otherwise specified |
| 141.6 | tip of tongue |
| 141.7 | border(s) of tongue |
| 141.8 | "anterior two-thirds," not otherwise specified |
| 141.9 | tongue, unspecified |
| | C. Salivary gland |
| 142.0 | parotid gland |
| 142.1 | submaxillary gland |
| 142.2 | sublingual gland |
| 142.9 | "salivary gland," not otherwise specified (<u>not</u> to include salivary gland type tumors in sites other than the major salivary glands; code salivary gland type tumors in other sites to the site where they appear.) |
| | D. Mouth |
| | 1. Floor of mouth (including lower gum) |
| 143.1 | floor of mouth |
| 143.2 | lower gum (gingiva covering lower alveolar ridge) |
| 143.5 | "book-leaf" neoplasm |
| 143.9 | both 143.1 and 143.2 - cannot determine which is site of origin |
| | 2. Other mouth and mouth, not otherwise specified |
| 144.1 | buccal mucosa |
| 144.2 | upper gum (gingiva covering upper alveolar ridge) |
| 144.3 | gum, not otherwise specified (gingiva not specified as upper or lower) |
| 144.4 | hard palate |
| 144.5 | soft palate, including uvula |
| 144.6 | palate, not otherwise specified |
| 144.7 | retromolar trigone (area of mucous membrane posterior to lower alveolar ridge and not coded in 143.1 or 143.2) |
| 144.9 | mouth, not otherwise specified |
| | E. Pharynx |
| | 1. Oral mesopharynx |
| 145.0 | tonsil, including fossa but excluding pillars |
| 145.1 | tonsillar pillars (pillars of fauces) |
| 145.2 | lateral wall |

| ICD CODE | SITE DESIGNATION |
|---|---|
| 145.3 | anterior wall (including lingual surface of epiglottis) |
| 145.4 | posterior wall |
| 145.5 | wall, not otherwise specified |
| 145.6 | vallecula |
| 145.7 | branchial cleft |
| 145.9 | oral mesopharynx, not otherwise specified |
| 146.- | 2. Nasopharynx (wall) |
| | 3. Hypopharynx |
| 147.0 | postcricoid region |
| 147.1 | pyriform fossa |
| 147.8 | other specified parts (posterior pharyngeal wall) |
| 147.9 | hypopharynx, not otherwise specified |
| 148.- | 4. Pharynx, not otherwise specified |
| | II. Digestive System |
| | A. Esophagus |
| 150.1 | upper third (cervical) |
| 150.2 | junction of upper and middle thirds |
| 150.3 | middle third (thoracic) at level of aortic arch |
| 150.4 | junction of middle and lower thirds |
| 150.5 | lower third (distal), including "abdominal esophagus" |
| 150.6 | cardio-esophageal junction (if not specified whether stomach or esophagus is the primary site, code here if <u>not</u> adenocarcinoma) |
| 150.9 | esophagus, not otherwise specified |
| | B. Stomach |
| 151.0 | cardio-esophageal junction, including cardia (if junction is not specified whether stomach or esophagus is the primary site, code here if adeno-carcinoma of any type) |
| 151.1 | fundus |
| | body |
| 151.2 | greater curvature of body; greater curvature, not otherwise specified |
| 151.3 | lesser curvature of body |
| 151.4 | body, not otherwise specified |
| | antrum and pylorus (including prepylorus) |
| 151.5 | greater curvature of antrum |
| 151.6 | lesser curvature of antrum |
| 151.7 | antrum, not otherwise specified; pylorus, not otherwise specified; prepylorus |
| 151.8 | lesser curvature, not otherwise specified |
| 151.9 | stomach, not otherwise specified |
| | C. Small intestine including duodenum |
| 152.0 | duodenum |
| 152.1 | jejunum |

| ICD CODE | SITE DESIGNATION |
|---|---|
| 152.2 | ileum excluding ileocecal valve |
| 152.9 | "small intestine," not otherwise specified |
| | D. Large intestine except rectum |
| 153.0 | ascending colon |
| 153.1 | transverse colon, including hepatic and splenic flexures |
| 153.2 | descending colon |
| 153.3 | sigmoid colon, excluding recto-sigmoid colon and junction |
| 153.4 | cecum, including caput coli |
| 153.5 | appendix |
| 153.6 | ileocecum; ileocecal valve |
| 153.7 | familial polyposis with at least one malignancy (any part of colon) |
| 153.9 | large intestine, not otherwise specified; colon, not otherwise specified |
| | E. Rectum |
| 154.1 | peri-anal skin — If "skin of anus," not otherwise specified, consult pathologist for better definition. Otherwise, assign squamous and basal to 154.1 and 154.2 |
| 154.2 | anal canal, anus, anal mucosa |
| 154.3 | rectum |
| 154.4 | rectosigmoid (specified), including junction |
| 154.7 | cloacogenic zone |
| 154.9 | ano-rectal region, not otherwise specified |
| | F. Liver, gallbladder, biliary passages (liver/biliary passages) |
| 155.1 | gallbladder |
| 155.2 | ampulla of Vater |
| 155.3 | extrahepatic bile ducts, including common duct |
| | liver and intrahepatic bile ducts |
| 155.5 | right lobe of liver |
| 155.6 | left lobe of liver |
| 155.7 | liver, not otherwise specified, including "both lobes," not specified which lobe was origin |
| | G. Pancreas |
| 157.1 | head |
| 157.8 | body; tail |
| 157.9 | pancreas, not otherwise specified |
| | III. Respiratory System |
| | A. Nose, nasal cavities, middle ear, accessory sinuses (nose/sinuses) |
| 160.0 | internal nose and nasal cavities, including nose, not otherwise specified, and nasal septum |

| ICD CODE | SITE DESIGNATION |
|---|---|
| 160.1 | eustachian tube and middle ear |
| 160.2 | maxillary sinus, maxillary antrum, antrum of Highmore |
| 160.3 | ethmoid sinus |
| 160.4 | sphenoid sinus |
| 160.5 | frontal sinus |
| 160.9 | "accessory sinus," not otherwise specified; paranasal sinus not otherwise specified |

Note: Excluded from this group of codes are the following sites: skin of nose; bone of nose; cartilage of ear; skin of ear, not otherwise specified; external auricular canal

| | |
|---|---|
| | B. Larynx |
| 161.1 | supraglottic region [epiglottis (laryngeal surface and not otherwise specified); arytenoids; false vocal cords; ventricular bands; ventricular cavities] |
| 161.2 | glottic region (glottis, true vocal cords) |
| 161.3 | subglottic region |
| 161.9 | larynx, not otherwise specified |
| | C. Bronchus, trachea, pleura, lung (lung/bronchus) |
| 162.0 | trachea, including carina |
| 162.2 | pleura |
| 162.3 | main bronchus (specified), including hilus |
| 162.4 | upper lobe, including segmental bronchus (code Pancoast's tumor here) |
| 162.5 | middle lobe or lingula, including segmental bronchus |
| 162.6 | lower lobe, including segmental bronchus |
| 162.9 | lung, not otherwise specified; bronchus, not otherwise specified |
| | D. Other respiratory organs<br>Mediastinum and respiratory, not otherwise specified |
| 164.1 | mediastinum |
| 164.9 | "respiratory organs," not otherwise specified |
| | IV. Breast and Reproductive Organs |
| 170.- | A. Breast, excluding skin of breast |
| 171.- | B. Cervix uteri |
| 171.1 | cervical stump |
| 172.- | C. Corpus uteri, including fundus uteri, endometrium |
| 174.- | D. Uterus, not otherwise specified |
| 175.- | E. Ovary |

| ICD CODE | SITE DESIGNATION |
|---|---|
| | F. Other and unspecified female genital organs |
| 173.- | 1. female trophoblastic tumors, including chorionepithelioma (excludes malignant fibroid tumors which are coded usually to 172.-) |
| 175.1 | 2. fallopian tube and broad ligament |
| 175.9 | 3. uterine adnexa, not otherwise specified |
| 176.0 | 4. vulva, including clitoris; labia; Bartholin's gland; skin of vulva; and also "pudendum" |
| 176.1 | 5. vagina |
| 176.7 | 6. other specified female genital sites, including parametrium |
| 176.9 | 7. "female genital organ," not otherwise specified |
| 177.- | G. Prostate |
| 178.- | H. Testis (including male chorionepithelioma if no primary site is stated) |
| | I. Other and unspecified male genital organs |
| 179.0 | 1. penis, including glans, prepuce, skin of penis |
| 179.1 | 2. skin of scrotum; scrotum, not otherwise specified |
| 179.2 | 3. tunica vaginalis |
| 179.3 | 4. epididymis |
| 179.7 | 5. other specified male genital sites, including seminal vesicle, spermatic cord, vas deferens, ductus deferens |
| 179.9 | 6. "male genital organ," not otherwise specified |
| | V. Urinary System |
| | A. Kidney/ureter |
| 180.0 | kidney parenchyma |
| 180.1 | renal pelvis |
| 180.2 | ureter |
| 180.9 | kidney, not otherwise specified |
| | B. Bladder |
| 181.0 | floor of bladder, base, trigone (not including areas of any orifice) |
| 181.1 | areas of ureter orifices |
| 181.2 | neck of bladder, including area of urethral orifice |
| 181.3 | fundus, vertex, dome, roof (not including area of any orifice) |
| 181.4 | wall (any and not otherwise specified) with no mention of orifice |

| ICD CODE | SITE DESIGNATION |
|---|---|
| 181.7 | abnormality as primary site of tumor (i.e., diverticulum, extrophy) |
| 181.8 | lesions in more than one sub-site 181.0-181.7 at first episode |
| 181.9 | bladder, not otherwise specified |
| | VI. Lymphatic and Hematopoietic Tissues |
| | A. Lymphomas and myeloma |
| 100.0 | 1. reticulum-cell sarcoma |
| 100.1 | 2. lymphosarcoma |
| 100.2 | 3. other primary malignant neoplasms of lymphoid tissue |
| 101.- | 4. Hodgkin's disease |
| 102.0 | 5. giant follicular lymphoma (Brill-Symmers' disease) |
| 102.1 | 6. other forms of lymphoma or reticulosis, not elsewhere classifiable |
| 103.- | 7. multiple myeloma |
| | B. Leukemias |
| 104.0 | 1. lymphatic leukemia, chronic or unspecified |
| 104.1 | 2. myeloid leukemia, chronic or unspecified |
| 104.2 | 3. monocytic leukemia (any) |
| 104.3 | 4. acute leukemia not coded to 104.2, 104.8, 104.9 (includes acute leukemia, not otherwise specified) |
| 104.4 | 5. other or unspecified leukemia not classifiable as acute |
| 104.5 | 6. acute erythremia (Di Guglielmo's disease) |
| 104.7 | 7. erythroleukemia |
| 104.8 | 8. acute lymphatic leukemia |
| 104.9 | 9. acute myeloid leukemia not identifiable as monocytic |
| | VII. Remaining and Ill-Defined Sites |
| | A. Malignant melanoma of skin |
| 190.0 | lip |
| 190.1 | eyelid, including canthi |
| 190.2 | external ear and auricular canal |
| 190.3 | other and unspecified parts of face |
| 190.4 | scalp and skin of neck |
| 190.5 | trunk, including skin of breast but excluding peri-anal skin, anus, and skin of genital organs |
| 190.6 | skin of upper limb excluding skin of shoulder |
| 190.7 | skin of lower limb including skin of hip |
| 190.8 | lesions in more than one sub-site 190.0-190.7 at first episode |

| ICD CODE | SITE DESIGNATION |
|---|---|
| 190.9 | melanoma of skin, not otherwise specified, including melanoma, not otherwise specified, of unspecified site |
| 192.- | B. Eye, including optic nerve but excluding skin and cartilage of eyelid |
| | C. Nervous system |
| 193.0 | 1. brain and cranial nerves, excluding optic nerve |
| 193.1 | 2. spinal cord |
| 193.3 | 3. peripheral nerves |
| 193.4 | 4. sympathetic nervous system, including retroperitoneal neuroblastoma |
| 193.5 | 5. cranial meninges except of optic nerve |
| 193.6 | 6. spinal meninges |
| 193.7 | 7. meninges, not otherwise specified |
| 193.9 | 8. unspecified nervous system site |
| 194.- | D. Thyroid gland |
| | E. Bone |
| 196.0 | skull and bones of face, including maxilla |
| 196.1 | lower jaw bone, including mandible |
| 196.2 | vertebral column, excluding sacrum and coccyx |
| 196.3 | ribs, sternum, and clavicle |
| 196.4 | scapula and long bones of upper limb (humerus, radius, ulna) |
| 196.5 | bones of fingers, hand, and wrist |
| 196.6 | pelvic bones, sacrum, coccyx (ilium, ischium, pubis, sacral vertebra) |
| 196.7 | long bones of lower limb (femur, fibula, tibia) |
| 196.8 | bones of toes, foot, ankle, knee cap |
| 196.9 | "bone," not otherwise specified |
| | F. Connective and soft tissue (soft tissue) |
| 197.0 | head, face, and neck |
| 197.1 | trunk, including heart |
| 197.2 | upper limb, including shoulder |
| 197.3 | lower limb, including hip |
| 197.4 | retroperitoneum, including retroperitoneal tumor, not otherwise specified, but excluding retroperitoneal neuroblastoma |
| 197.9 | connective tissue, site unspecified; muscle, not otherwise specified |
| | G. Other and unspecified sites |
| 105.- | 1. mycosis fungoides |
| 158.- | 2. peritoneum excluding "retroperitoneum," but including omentum, mesentery, mesocolon |

| ICD CODE | SITE DESIGNATION |
|---|---|
| | 3. Unspecified digestive organs |
| 159.1 | "intestinal tract," not otherwise specified |
| 159.9 | "digestive organs," not otherwise specified; "digestive tract," not otherwise specified |
| | 4. Other urinary organs |
| 182.0 | urethra |
| 182.1 | urachus |
| 183.9 | 5. lower genitourinary tract, not otherwise specified |
| | 6. Other endocrine glands |
| 195.0 | suprarenal gland (adrenal gland) |
| 195.1 | parathyroid gland |
| 195.2 | thymus |
| 195.3 | pituitary gland and craniopharyngeal duct |
| 195.4 | pineal gland |
| 195.5 | chemoreceptor gland or organ, including carotid body, aortic body, glomus jugulare, glomus ciliare, glomus intravagale, and chemodectoma with site not specified |
| 195.7 | other endocrine gland, not elsewhere classifiable |
| | 7. Ill-defined sites |
| 199.- | primary site completely unspecified or not specified enough to be classified to more specific code (including carcinomatosis, not otherwise specified; sarcomatosis, not otherwise specified; generalized, not otherwise specified, etc.) |

# Epilogue

*"What is past is prologue."*
*SHAKESPEARE, The Tempest,*
*Act II, Scene I, Line 261*

In the preface to this volume we addressed the question of why one should study patients with multiple primary cancer and have, hopefully, justified the usefulness of such an endeavor. As noted in Chapter 1, there have been many investigations of this phenomenon, one of the most complete being MOERTEL's study published in 1966 as volume 7 of Recent Results in Cancer Research. An equally valid parallel question is why carry out another study of multiple primary cancer as represented by the present volume.

On closer inspection, however, the scope and approach of the studies are quite different. The characteristics of these two investigations are contrasted in Table 139.

MOERTEL's analysis is based on the experience of patients with malignant neoplasms seen at the Mayo Clinic and its affiliated hospitals during a ten-year period. Only patients with histologically proven malignancies were accepted. The clinical, surgical, and pathologic records of these individuals were carefully reviewed by MOERTEL to verify the presence of any reported multiple primary malignant neoplasms. In equivocal cases, tissue specimens were re-evaluated. Where doubt remained with regards to distinguishing between a metastatic lesion and a new primary malignant neoplasm, the tumor was excluded. Among a total of 37,580 patients under observation, 1,153 subsequent primary neoplasms were diagnosed. This figure excludes multiple primaries discovered at the same time as the initial malignant neoplasm.

MOERTEL's data have certain distinct advantages as well as some definite limitations. The importance of carefully reviewing all reported cases of multiple primary cancer, especially when done by a single individual, cannot be overemphasized. Whatever biases may exist on the part of the reviewer are at least consistent biases which are applied equally to all the cases. However, not all malignant neoplasms are microscopically confirmed. For example, a glioblastoma because of its critical anatomic location may never be biopsied, and if the patient dies, an autopsy examination may be refused. One must weigh the advantages and disadvantages of excluding such cases from consideration.

By restricting one's analysis to the experience of a single medical institution one is assured of some reasonable degree of uniformity in the collection of clinical data as well as relatively easy access to records and tissue specimens. However, such an approach, based on a selected segment of the population, poses certain limitations on the usefulness and extent of the tabulations which are possible. The problem is that cancer patients seen at the Mayo Clinic and its affiliated institutions may not be representative of all cancer patients in the general population. Thus, one must use great caution in attempting to

Table 139. Comparison of Mayo Clinic Series and Present Connecticut Series

| | Mayo Clinic Series | Connecticut Series |
|---|---|---|
| Type of Study | Descriptive | Analytic |
| Group Under Observation | Patients with malignant neoplasms evaluated at Mayo Clinic and affiliated hospitals | All Connecticut residents with diagnosis of malignant neoplasm admitted to hospital in Connecticut or neighboring state, or who have cancer listed on death certificate |
| Population From Which Observed Group is Derived | Unknown | Population of Connecticut |
| Years Surveyed | 1944-53, inclusive | 1935-64, inclusive |
| Exclusion of Cases | Multiple epitheliomas of skin; non-histologically confirmed malignant neoplasms | Non-melanotic skin cancer |
| Review of Reported Cases | Author's review of clinical, surgical, and pathologic records (in doubtful cases tissue specimens were also reviewed) | No general review of cases reported to the Connecticut Tumor Registry |
| Number of Patients With Index Malignant Neoplasm Observed for Development of Another Malignant Neoplasm | 37,580 | 121,460 |
| Number of Additional Malignant Tumors Diagnosed After the Index Malignant Neoplasm | 1,153 | 5,022 |

generalize from the findings of a study based on individuals seen at a given medical institution. Analyzing the experience of a single clinic or hospital poses an additional restriction in that the population from which this group of patients is derived, remains largely unknown. One is confined to a descriptive study of the observed characteristics in the group of patients under care. When the population from which these patients are derived is unknown, it is difficult to select a control group against which to compare these observations. Although one can describe the number of multiple primaries, their anatomic site, the time interval between tumors, the age of the patients, etc., it is impossible to determine whether these observations might be expected based on the experience of patients with a single primary cancer.

The investigation of the Connecticut Tumor Registry's data was designed as an analytic study in which the observed characteristics of patients developing multiple primary cancer can be compared to a control group of patients developing a single cancer. This enables one to determine whether individuals with one cancer are at increased, decreased, or unchanged risk of developing a subsequent primary cancer. This is possible only because the incidence rates used to calculate the expected number of multiple primary cancers are obtained from the same population yielding the first primary cancers. The Connecticut Tumor Registry has sufficiently large experience in terms of the size of its population base and the length of time this population has been under observation to allow meaningful comparisons between the observed and expected number of second primary cancers by anatomic site of the tumors, time interval between the tumors, and sex of the patient.

In contrast to MOERTEL's report, the Connecticut tabulations presented in this monograph are analytic in their consideration of the multiple primary cancer problem. The group under observation consisted of all Connecticut residents with a diagnosis of malignant neoplasm (excluding non-melanotic skin cancer) who were admitted to a hospital in Connecticut or neighboring states, or who had cancer listed on their death certificate. Such cases are routinely submitted to the Connecticut Tumor Registry which served as the data resource. In this investigation the reporting physician determined whether a tumor was a metastatic lesion or a new primary cancer. Although selected reviews were possible, it was impractical with regards to both time and expense for a single individual to re-evaluate the several thousand clinical and pathologic records or tissue specimens which are kept at the various participating hospitals in Connecticut and neighboring states. This situation creates the type of problem recognized earlier in this century by the British statistician, Sir JOSIAH STAMP, who wrote: "The government [statisticians] are very keen on amassing statistics -- they collect them, add them, raise them to the nth power, take the cube root and prepare wonderful diagrams. But what you must never forget is that every one of those figures comes in the first instance from the ... village watchman, who puts down what he damn pleases" (STAMP, 1929). In the case of Connecticut, the reporting physicians represent our village watchmen. Consequently, the reader must remain cautious in drawing conclusions from the tabulations derived from the Connecticut Tumor Registry. Histologic verification is extremely important. Corroboration from other investigations becomes essential. Among the 121,460 patients with a first primary malignancy, 5,022 subsequent primary cancers were reported.

It is obvious from these discussions that the ideal epidemiologic study of multiple primary cancers does not yet exist. MOERTEL's analysis is restricted to reporting observed characteristics of the Mayo patients and is hampered by the lack of an identifiable population from which these patients are derived. The Connecticut study is based on a well-defined population, but the diagnostic validity of the reported cases has not been systematically verified by a single reviewer. To do so, would at the present time, require an inordinate expenditure of time and money. However, the Connecticut material represents the highest quality data currently available on a large, well-defined population under observation for many years. The ideal study will be approached only when all cases of multiple primary cancer reported to the registry are routinely reviewed and have microscopic confirmation.

In the meantime, the tabulations assembled in this monograph should not be thought of as the concluding chapter in some hypothetical, definitive work on multiple primary cancer. Rather, these data should be regarded as a preface upon which to formulate more refined studies to be the subject of future volumes.

## Reference

STAMP, J.: Some Economic Factors in Modern Life, London: P.S. King and Son, Ltd. 1929, pp. 258-259

# Subject Index


acoustic neuroma, 23
adenomatosis, anatomic sites paired with, 23, 26
adrenal cortex tumors, primary, 23
alcohol, digestive tract cancer and, 34, 48
anal cancer, metastases of, 68
anatomic sites, international classification of disease by, 155-163

biliary passage cancer, 158
- metastases of, 68
- neoplasms associated with, 63-64
bladder cancers, 160-161
- metastases of, 115
- neoplasms associated with, 112-114, 143, 144, 146
- primary
-- lung cancer and, 23, 24
-- multiple 9, 21
- secondary 9, 10, 13
- smoking and, 70, 109
bone cancers, 162
- metastases of, 140
- neoplasms associated with, 133-134, 143
- secondary, 21, 124
brain tumors
- breast cancer and, 23, 24-25, 124
- in Turcot's syndrome, 23
- neoplasms associated with, 129-130
breast cancers, 159
- colon cancer and, 82
- metastases of, 107
- neoplasms associated with, 80-107, 143, 144, 146
-- table, 85-87
- person-years of observation of, 16
- primary, multiple tumors and, 6, 9, 11, 12, 13, 23
- salivary gland cancers with, 28, 34
- secondary, 9, 10, 11, 13, 20
- site-group combinations with, 23, 24-25, 106
- soft tissue tumors following, 27, 82-83
bronchial cancers, 159
- neoplasms associated with, 75-76, 143, 144, 146
- primary, 23
- secondary, 13
buccal cavity cancers, 48, 69, 155
- metastatic sites for, 46
- primary, 11
-- multiple, 6
-- neoplasms associated with, 33-46

cecum cancer, primary, multiple tumors and, 10
cerebellum, hemangiomas of, 23
cervical cancer, smoking and, 83
cervix cancers, 159
- metastases of, 107
- neoplasms associated with, 88-90, 143
- primary, 13
-- multiple, 9, 12, 20
-- secondary, 20
-- sites related to, 23, 26, 83
chemical carcinogens, multiple primary neoplasms from, 23
chemotherapy, in etiology of primary multiple tumors, 23, 27
cigarette smoking, see smoking
colon cancer
- breast cancer and, 82

- female genital cancer and, 23, 48
- infertility and, 25, 82
- metastases of, 68
- neoplasms associated with, 57-59, 143, 144, 146
- primary, 4, 20
-- multiple tumors and, 10, 12, 20, 23
- secondary, 10, 11, 12, 13, 20
- urinary tract cancer with, 49
colon tumors, in Turcot's syndrome, 23
computer, use in primary tumor data analysis, 4
Connecticut Tumor Registry
- data in, 4-5
- description of, 4, 15
- summary of results of, 141-146
connective tissue tumors, 162
cyclophosphamide, myeloma treatment by, carcinomas following, 23

digestive system cancers
- primary, 10
-- multiple tumors and, 4, 10, 11
-- neoplasms following, 47-68
- secondary, 9
digestive tract cancers, 157-158
- neoplasms associated with, 33
- site-group pairs in, 67
dog, primary cancers in, 6

ear cancers, neoplasms associated with, 71-72
endocrine factors, in etiology of primary multiple neoplasms, 23
endocrine gland tumors, 163
endometrial cancer
- infertility and, 25, 81
- intestinal cancer and, 48
endometrium cancer
- primary, multiple tumors and, 9, 10
ependymoma, 23
epidermal cysts, in Gardner's syndrome, 23
esophageal cancers, 157
- metastases of, 68
- neoplasms associated with, 50-51, 146
- primary, 20, 24
-- multiple, 48
- secondary, 13, 20
- subsequent neoplasms following, 143, 144
eye tumors, 124, 162
- metastases of, 140
- neoplasms associated with, 127-128, 143, 144, 146
- secondary, 21

fibromas, in Gardner's syndrome, 23

gallbladder cancers, 158
Gardner's syndrome, tumors paired with, 23, 124
genetic factors, in etiology of primary multiple tumors, 23, 24, 26
genital system tumors, see also individual organs)
genital system index tumors
- in females, 4
-- multiple tumors and, 10
genital system primary tumors
- second primary cancers and, 4
genital system tumors
- secondary, 9

hematopoietic tissue tumors, 161
- neoplasms associated with, 116-122
high-risk cancer patients, identification of, 3
Hodgkin's disease
- as primary cancer, multiple tumors and, 9, 11
- neoplasms following treatment for, 23, 27, 28
hypernephroma, 23

immune defects, in etiology of primary multiple tumors, 23, 27
infertility, endometrial cancer and, 25, 81, 82
intestinal tumors, primary, 23

kidney cancers, 160
- metastases of, 115
- neoplasms associated with, 110-111, 143, 144, 146
- primary, multiple, 21
- secondary, 12, 13, 21, 83

large intestine cancers, 157
- primary, multiple tumors and, 10
- secondary, 10
laryngeal cancers, 159
- neoplasms associated with, 73-74, 143
- primary, 20, 24
- secondary, 20
leukemia(s), 160
- as primary cancer, 21
-- multiple tumors and, 9, 11
- following multiple myeloma, 23
- immunodeficiency and, 27
- neoplasms associated with, 47, 82-83, 116-122, 143, 144, 146
-- table of, 120-121
- thyroid cancer and, 124
lip cancers, 155
- primary, multiple, 7-9, 11, 12, 20
- subsequent neoplasms following, 35-36, 143, 144, 146
lipomas, in Gardner's syndrome, 23, 26
liver cancers, 158
- metastases of, 68
- neoplasms associated with, 63-64
- primary, 20
- secondary, 20
lung cancers, 159
- neoplasms associated with, 75-76, 143, 144, 146
- primary, 20
-- multiple, 20
- secondary, 13
lung cancer primary
- bladder cancer and, 23, 24
- scrotal cancer and, 23
lymphangiosarcoma, following surgery for breast cancer, 23, 82
lymphatic leukemia, and immune defects, 23
lymphatic tissue tumors, 161
- metastases of, 122
- neoplasms associated with, 116-122
lymphomas, 161
- neoplasms associated with, 118-119, 143
- primary multiple, 21
lymphoreticular tumors, immunodeficiency and, 27
lymphosarcoma, as primary cancer, multiple tumors, and, 9
male genital organs, neoplasms associated with, 102-105, 143
malignancy, definition of, 155
malignant melanoma, 5, 161-162
- metastases of, 140
- neoplasms associated with, 125-126, 139, 143, 144, 146
- primary, 12, 123
marital status, breast cancer and, 24-25, 48
mediastinal cancers, 159
- neoplasms associated with, 77-78
melanoma, primary, multiple, 21
meningiomas
- primary, 13
-- breast cancer and, 23, 124
metastases
- of buccal cavity tumors, 46
- of digestive tract tumors, 68
- of lymphatic tissue tumors, 122
- of reproductive organ cancers, 107
- of respiratory system cancers, 79
- primary tumors and, 1
-- criteria, 4
mineral oil, cancers associated with, 23, 24
mouth cancers, 156
- primary, 20
-- multiple, 11, 12, 20, 24
- prostatic cancer with, 33
- secondary, 12, 20
- subsequent neoplasms following, 41-43, 143, 144, 146
multiple myeloma, leukemias following treatment for, 23, 27
myelomas, 161
- as primary cancer, multiple tumors and, 9, 11
- neoplasms associated with, 118-119, 143

nasal cavities
- primary cancers of, 11, 20, 158-159
-- multiple, 20, 71-72
- secondary, 20
- subsequent neoplasms to, 143
nasopharynx, primary cancers of, 11
nervous system tumors, 162

- neoplasms associated with, 129-130, 143, 145
- primary, 4
-- multiple, 21
- secondary, 21
neurofibromas, multiple, 23
nose cancers, 158-159
- neoplasms associated with, 71-72
nutritional factors, in etiology of primary multiple neoplasms, 23, 24

osteomas, in Gardner's syndrome, 23
osteosarcomas
- after radiation therapy, 23, 26-27
- primary, retinoblastomas and, 23
ovarian cancer, 159
- metastases of, 107
- neoplasms associated with, 95-96, 143, 144, 146
- primary, 12
-- multiple, 21
- secondary, 11, 12, 13, 20, 47

pancreatic cancers, 158
- metastases of, 68
- neoplasms associated with, 65-66, 143, 145
- primary, 20, 23
- secondary, 20, 47
paranasal sinus cancer, primary cancers of, 11
parathyroid tumors, 23
- primary, 23, 26
- sites associated with, 27
penile cancer, 160
- metastases of, 107
peritoneum cancer, after other index tumors, 9
person-years
- breast cancer observation by, 16-17
- definition of, 29
pharyngeal cancers, 155-157
- neoplasms associated with, 33-46, 146
-- table of, 44-45
- primary, 11, 20
-- multiple, 11, 12, 20
- secondary, 13, 20, 47
- subsequent neoplasms following, 143, 144
pheochromocytoma, 23
- anatomic sites paired with, 23
pituitary tumors, primary, site-group pairs with, 23, 26
Poisson distribution, of subsequent primary cancers, 18
primary tumors
- criteria for, 1
- metastasis compared to, criteria, 4
- multiple
-- non-simultaneously diagnosed, 22-32
-- simultaneously diagnosed, 19-21
- simultaneous 1
-- summary of, 5-13
prostate cancers, 160
- leukemia and, 83, 116-117
- metastases of, 107
- mouth cancer with, 33
- neoplasms associated with, 99-101, 143, 144, 146
- primary, multiple tumors and, 9, 21
- respiratory tract cancer and, 69
- secondary, 9, 12, 21, 47

radiation, multiple primary cancers and, 23, 26
rectal cancers, 158
- after radiation therapy, 23
- metastases of, 68
- multiple tumors and, 10, 12, 20
- neoplasms associated with, 48, 60-62, 143, 144, 146
- primary, 4, 13, 20
- secondary, 12, 13, 20
rectosigmoid junction cancer, primary, multiple tumors and, 10
reproductive organ cancers, 159-160
- neoplasms associated with, 80-107
respiratory tract cancers, 158-159
- metastases of, 19
- neoplasms associated with, 33, 69-79, 143-146
- primary cancers of, 47
-- multiple, 11
- smoking and, 69-70
retina, hemangiomas of, 23
retinoblastoma, 23
- neoplasms associated with, 23, 24, 27, 123-124

salivary gland cancers, 156
- primary, 20, 23
-- multiple tumors and, 10, 12
- subsequent neoplasms following, 23, 28, 34, 39-40, 143
sarcomas, metastases of, 140
scrotal cancer, primary, lung cancer and, 23, 24
site-group pairs, in multiple malignancies, 23
skin cancers
- from immune defects, 23, 28
- leukemia and, 117
skin primary cancers
- data registry of, 5-13
- multiple, 6-13
small intestine cancers, 157-158
- metastases of, 68
- neoplasms associated with, 47, 55-56, 143, 144, 146
- primary, 20
- secondary, 12, 13, 20
smoking, multiple primary cancers and, 23, 24, 47, 48, 69, 70
soft tissue tumors, 162
- neoplasms associated with, 135-136, 143, 144, 146
- secondary, 21, 48, 82
squamous cell carcinomas, multiple primaries of, 11
statistics, of subsequent primary cancer incidence, 18
stomach cancers, 157
- metastases of, 68
- neoplasms associated with, 48, 52-54, 143, 145
- primary, 13, 20
-- multiple, 10, 20
- secondary, 20
surgery, in etiology of primary multiple tumors, 23
survival intervals, 15-16

thymoma, and immune defects, 23, 27-28
thyroid gland cancers, 162
- leukemia and, 124
- metastases of, 140
- neoplasms associated with, 131-132, 143, 144, 146
- primary, 12, 23
- secondary, 21
tobacco, multiple primary neoplasms and, 23, 24
tongue cancers, 155-156
- primary, 20
- secondary, 20
- subsequent neoplasms following 37-38, 143, 144
tumor registries, importance of, 3
Turcot's syndrome, tumors paired with, 23
testicular cancers, 160
- neoplasms associated with, 83-84, 102-103, 107, 143, 144, 146
- primary, multiple, 20, 21

ureter cancers, 160
- metastases of, 115
- neoplasms associated with, 110-111, 143, 144, 146
- primary, multiple, 21
- secondary, 12, 13, 83
urinary system tumors, 160-161, 163
- neoplasms associated with, 108-115
uterine cancers, 159
- colon cancer with, 23
- metastases of, 107
- neoplasms associated with, 24-25, 91-94, 143, 144, 146
- primary, 13
-- multiple, 8-9, 12, 20
- secondary, 11

von Hippel-Lindau disease, primary tumors of, anatomic sites paired with, 23
von Recklinghausen's disease, primary tumors of, anatomic sites paired with, 23

# Recent Results in Cancer Research

Sponsored by the Swiss League against Cancer. Editor in Chief: P. Rentchnick, Genève

**For information about Vols. 1—9, please contact your bookseller or Springer-Verlag.**

10 NELSON, R. S.: Radioactive Phosphorus in the Diagnosis of Gastrointestinal Cancer.

11 FREEMAN, R. G. and J. M. KNOX: Treatment of Skin Cancer.

12 LYNCH, H. T.: Hereditary Factors in Carcinoma.

13 Tumours in Children, 2nd Edition. Edited by H. B. MARSDEN and J. K. STEWARD.

14 ODARTCHENKO, N.: Production Cellulaire Erythropoïétique.

15 SOKOLOFF, B.: Carcinoid and Serotonin.

16 JACOBS, M. L.: Malignant Lymphomas and Their Management.

17 Normal and Malignant Cell Growth. Edited by R. J. M. FRY, M. L. GRIEM, and W. H. KIRSTEN (Symposium).

18 ANGLESIO, E.: The Treatment of Hodgkin's Disease.

19 BANNASCH, P.: The Cytoplasm of Hepatocytes during Carcinogenesis. Electron- and Lightmicroscopical Investigations of the Nitrosomorpholine-intoxicated Rat Liver.

20 Rubidomycin. A new Agent against Cancer. Edited by J. BERNARD, R. PAUL, M. BOIRON, C. JACQUILLAT, and R. MARAL.

21 Scientific Basis of Cancer Chemotherapy. Edited by G. MATHÉ (Symposium).

22 KOLDOVSKÝ, P.: Tumor Specific Transplantation Antigen.

23 FUCHS, W. A., J. W. DAVIDSON, and H. W. FISCHER: Lymphography in Cancer. With contributions by G. JANTET and H. RÖSLER.

24 HAYWARD, J.: Hormones und Human Breast Cancer. An Account of 15 Years Study.

25 ROY-BURMAN, P.: Analogues of Nucleic Acid Components. Mechanisms of Action.

26 Tumors of the Liver. Edited by G. T. PACK and A. H. ISLAMI.

27 SZYMENDERA, J.: Bone Mineral Metabolism in Cancer.

28 MEEK, E. S.: Antitumour and Antiviral Substances of Natural Origin.

29 Aseptic Environments and Cancer Treatment. Edited by G. MATHÉ (Symposium).

30 Advances in the Treatment of Acute (Blastic) Leukemias. Edited by G. MATHÉ (Symposium).

31 DENOIX, P.: Treatment of Malignant Breast Tumors. Indications and Results.

32 NELSON, R. S.: Endoscopy in Gastric Cancer.

33 Experimental and Clinical Effects of L-Asparaginase. Edited by E. GRUNDMANN and H. F. OETTGEN (Symposium).

34 Chemistry and Biological Actions of 4-Nitroquinolin 1-Oxide. Edited by H. ENDO, T. ONO, and T. SUGIMURA.

35 PENN, I.: Malignant Tumors in Organ Transplant Recipients.

36 Current Concepts in the Management of Lymphoma and Leukemia. Edited by J. E. ULTMANN, M. L. GRIEM, W. H. KIRSTEN, and R. W. WISSLER (Symposium).

37 CHIAPPA, S., R. MUSUMECI, and C. USLENGHI: Endolymphatic Radiotherapy in Malignant Lymphomas. With contributions by G. BONADONNA, B. DAMASCELLI, G. FAVA, F. PIZZETTI, U. VERONESI.

38 KOLLER, P. C.: The Role of Chromosomes in Cancer Biology.

39 Current Problems in the Epidemiology of Cancer and Lymphomas. Edited by E. GRUNDMANN and H. TULINIUS (Symposium).

40 LANGLEY, F. A. and A. C. CROMPTON: Epithelial Abnormalities of the Cervix Uteri.

41 Tumours in a Tropical Country. A Survey of Uganda (1964—1968). Edited by A. C. TEMPLETON.

42 Breast Cancer: A Challenging Problem. Edited by M. L. GRIEM, E. V. JENSEN, J. E. ULTMANN, and R. W. WISSLER (Symposium).

43 Nomenclature, Methodology and Results of Clinical Trials in Acute Leukemias. Edited by G. MATHÉ, P. POUILLART, L. SCHWARZENBERG (Symposium).

44 Special Topics in Carcinogenesis. Edited by E. GRUNDMANN (Symposium).
45 KOLDOVSKÝ, P.: Carcinoembryonic Antigens.
46 Diagnosis and Therapy of Malignant Lymphoma. Edited by K. MUSSHOFF (Symposium).
47 Investigation and Stimulation of Immunity in Cancer Patients. Edited by G. MATHÉ and R. WEINER (Symposium).
48 Platinum Coordination Complexes in Cancer Chemotherapy. Edited by T. A. CONNORS and J. J. ROBERTS (Symposium).
49 Complications of Cancer Chemotherapy. Edited by G. MATHÉ and R. K. OLDHAM (Symposium).
50 Cancer Registry. Edited by E. GRUNDMANN and E. PEDERSEN (Symposium).
51 Gliomas. Current Concepts in Biology, Diagnosis and Therapy. Edited by J. HEKMATPANAH (Symposium).
52 The Ambivalence of Cytostatic Therapy. Edited by E. GRUNDMANN and R. GROSS (Symposium).
53 A. CLARYSSE, Y. KENIS, and G. MATHÉ: Cancer Chemotherapy.
54 Malignant Bone Tumors. Edited by E. GRUNDMANN.
55 MATHÉ, G.: Cancer Active Immunotherapy, Immunoprophylaxis, and Immunorestoration.
56 Lymphocytes, Macrophages, and Cancer. Edited by G. MATHÉ, I. FLORENTIN, and M.-C. SIMMLER (Symposium).
57 Breast Cancer: A Multidisciplinary Approach. Edited by G. ST. ARNEAULT, P. BAND, and L. ISRAËL (Symposium).
58 B. S. SCHOENBERG: Multiple Primary Malignant Neoplasms.
59 Selective Heat Sensitivity of Cancer Cells. Edited by A. ROSSI-FANELLI, R. CAVALIERE, B. MONDOVI, and G. MORICCA.
60 Tumors of the Male Genital System. Edited by E. GRUNDMANN and W. VAHLENSIECK (Symposium).

Special Supplement: Biology of Amphibian Tumors. Edited by M. MIZELL.

MIX
Papier aus verantwortungsvollen Quellen
Paper from responsible sources
FSC® C105338

If you have any concerns about our products,
you can contact us on
**ProductSafety@springernature.com**

In case Publisher is established outside the EU,
the EU authorized representative is:
**Springer Nature Customer Service Center GmbH**
**Europaplatz 3, 69115 Heidelberg, Germany**

Printed by Libri Plureos GmbH
in Hamburg, Germany